# Renal Diet Cookbook
# for Beginners 2020

**The Complete Renal Diet Guide with 4-Week Meal Plan to Managing
Chronic Kidney Disease**

**By Jacob Hoffman**

**Legal & Disclaimer**

The information contained in this book and its contents is not designed to replace or take the place of any form of medical or professional advice; and is not meant to replace the need for independent medical, financial, legal or other professional advice or services, as may be required. The content and information in this book has been provided for educational and entertainment purposes only.

The content and information contained in this book has been compiled from sources deemed reliable, and it is accurate to the best of the Author's knowledge, information, and belief. However, the Author cannot guarantee its accuracy and validity and cannot be held liable for any errors and/or omissions. Further, changes are periodically made to this book as and when needed. Where appropriate and/or necessary, you must consult a professional (including but not limited to your doctor, attorney, financial advisor or such other professional advisor) before using any of the suggested remedies, techniques, or information in this book.

You agree to accept all risks of using the information presented inside this book.

You agree that by continuing to read this book, where appropriate and/or necessary, you shall consult a professional (including but not limited to your doctor, attorney, or financial advisor or such other advisor as needed) before using any of the suggested remedies, techniques, or information in this book.

# Table of Contents

# Introduction

Have you been diagnosed with renal disease?

If yes, and your doctor has advised you some general diet guidelines on what to eat and what to avoid, maybe you still wondering about some details and recipes to try out while being on a renal diet.

When preparing your food, keep it less salty. Check the labels of the ingredients you are using. Checking labels will help you determine how much sodium you are consuming per day. There are many ingredients that have hidden sodium in them. Ingredients like baking powder, dressings, and processed powdered soup have hidden sodium.

Choosing fresh ingredients is always beneficial for renal patients. Eating seasonal food is an excellent way to find fresh vegetables and fruits. If you have to choose frozen food, go for the un-salty and unflavored kind. Canned food contains high potassium and high sodium liquid. Choose the ones that are clear.

When you go out to eat, choose renal friendly dishes. Order the drinks that have low sodium and low potassium. Clear ones are better than the colored ones. Choose healthy protein options. Divide your fluid into four different portions and drink them after certain hours to keep your thirst satisfied and without hurting the renal fluid limits.

My story with the renal diet started when a close friend of mine found out that she was suffering from a kidney disease. I didn't know much about kidney diseases and I was shocked when I discovered that my friend had to deal with a serious health condition. I never heard my dear friend complaining about her illness, neither was she afraid of it. Yet, I was committed to helping my friend lead an absolutely ordinary life and I accompanied her every time she would go to the hospital.

I had many conversations with other patients when my friend was seeing her doctor and many of them were on the verge of kidney failure. From the short time I spent with those patients, I learned that some of them used to work, but others gave up on living their normal lives. Their only hope was dialysis once, twice or thrice a week. I was surprised that many patients didn't know what caused their illness and they were hoping that they had the ability to rewind time so that they eat healthy and never harm their kidneys.

And on this framework, I take pride in writing this book and dedicate it to kidney disease patients. It is never too late to cope with your kidney disease and to avoid dialysis, especially if you detect it on time. I don't claim I have the same medical knowledge as doctors and specialists, but through this book, I am offering you the best renal diet book to guide you to a healthy body and kidneys. Indeed, the cornerstone of healthy kidneys lies in the diet you follow.

Following a renal diet can help limit the toxins and the waste in your body and can help your kidney function in a more effective way. So, if you suffer from any kidney disease, don't feel discouraged and don't lose hope because a simple diet can change your life for the better forever. And remember that any tiny change in your meal plan can help prevent dialysis.

# Chapter 1: The Detailed Information about Kidney Disease

Kidney disease or in other words "renal disease" and "kidney damage" is a health condition where the kidneys are unable to function in a healthy and proper manner. Chronic kidney disease is a slow-moving disease and does not cause the patient a lot of complaints in the initial stages. Chronic kidney disease includes a group of kidney diseases, in which case the renal function decreases for several years or decades. With the help of timely diagnosis and treatment, it can slow down and even stop the progression of kidney disease.

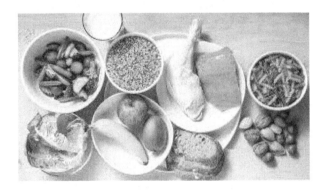

## How Kidneys Work and What Is Their Role in Our Systems?

Kidneys are vital organs located in our lower body backs (around the ribcage area) that are responsible for filtering out the toxins and junk out of our bloodstream through the urine. To preserve the balance in our systems, kidneys help regulate salts and minerals circulating in our bodies such as sodium, phosphorus, and potassium. Our kidneys also release hormonal compounds that help regulate blood pressure, build new red blood cells, and maintain healthy bones and connective tissue.

Anatomically, the kidneys are positioned in the abdomen, at the back, usually on both sides of the spine. The renal artery, which is a direct branch of the aorta supplies blood to the kidneys. Renal veins empty the blood from kidneys to the vena cava, then the heart. The word "renal" originated from the Latin word for kidney.

## Who Can Suffer From Chronic Kidney Disease?

Any person can develop the disease. The greatest risk of getting sick is in people who have one or more of the following risk factors:

- Diabetes
- High blood pressure
- Family members have previously had kidney disease
- Age over 50
- Long-term consumption of drugs that can damage the kidneys
- Overweight or obesity

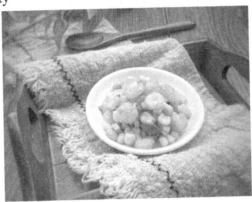

## Stages

Kidney disease, in this case, is a chronic condition (CKD) where the kidneys fail gradually to do their normal job. Chronic kidney disease typically develops in 5 stages. Each stage is measured by a formula called Glomerular Filtration Rate (GFR) which is calculated by several variables like age, race, gender, and the amount of serum creatinine in the urine. The higher this protein is in the system, the more progressed the stage of renal disease will be. Here is a brief snapshot of each stage.

Stage 1:considered the normal or high risk of developing CKD. The GFR falls > 90 mL/min.

Stage 2:considered as mild CKD. The GFR falls in the range of 60-89 mL/min.

Stage 3: Moderate CKD which ranges from 45-59 mL/min.

Stage 4:Severe Chronic Kidney disease. Rates fall between 15-29 mL/min.

Stage 5:Final/end-stage of the renal disease which calls for surgery or dialysis. Also called End-Stage Renal Disease (ESRD). The GFR levels, in this case, fall below 15 mL/min.

# Causes

Now, in regards to the actual causes or risk factors that may contribute to the formation of disease, studies have indicated the following conditions:

Diabetes. Diabetes is probably the No.1 cause of renal disease as the increased blood glucose in the bloodstream can actually ruin blood vessels inside the kidneys.

Heart disease. Heart disease has also been found to have a negative association with CKD. Those with chronic heart problems, in particular, have a higher probability of developing the renal disease as well.

Elevated blood pressure. Abnormally high blood pressure can ruin the delicate blood vessels inside the kidneys and make them function poorly as a result.

Genetic History of Renal Disease. If any of your family members and especially parents and grandparents have already developed the disease, there is a higher risk you are going to develop it too. If any of your family members has kidney disease, it would be wise to get tested too and encourage other family members to do the same.

In addition to the above common causes, autoimmune disorders like Lupus and nephrotic syndrome can increase the risk of developing renal disease. Also, urinary problems and certain medications e.g. diuretics or antibiotics, as well as illegal drugs, can also interfere with the normal function of the kidneys and cause damage. For this reason, it would be wise to consult your doctor and take drugs for other conditions e.g. diabetes that does not harm your kidneys as a side effect.

# Symptoms

The problem with the disease is that it often comes with little or no symptoms at all, especially during the first stages. You may experience the following symptoms, but these could also be a sign of another condition:

- Less frequent urination
- A very little amount of urine
- Sudden and unexplained pauses in breath
- Nausea
- Chest or back pain
- Drowsiness and dizziness
- Dry skin, itchy skin
- Fatigue/feeling tired more than before
- Confusion
- Loss of balance
- Muscle cramps especially at night
- Swelling in the face, ankles, feet, and hands
- Poor appetite

In extreme cases and stages e.g. renal failure, seizures and coma may also occur. However, it would be best for you to avoid looking solely for these symptoms and actually get tested to find out whether you have a chronic disease or not.

# Diagnosis

**Two Tests Are Can Be Prescribed By Your Family Doctor.**

1.  Blood test:glomerular filtration rate (GFR) and serum creatinine level. Creatinine is one of those end products of protein metabolism, the level in the blood depends on age, gender, muscle mass, nutrition, physical activity, on which foods before taking the sample (for example, a lot of meat was eaten), and some drugs. Creatinine is excreted from the body through the kidneys, and if the work of the kidneys slows down, the creatinine levels present in the blood plasma rises. Determining the level of creatinine alone is not sufficient for the diagnosis of chronic kidney disease since its value begins to exceed the upper limit of the norm only when GFR decreases by half. To calculate GFR, you include four parameters into your formula that take into account the creatinine reading, age, gender, and race of the patient. GFR shows at what level is the ability of the kidneys to filter. In the case of chronic kidney disease, the GFR indicator shows the stage of the severity of kidney disease.

2.  Urine analysis:the content of albumin in the urine is determined; also, the values of albumin and creatinine in the urine are determined by each other. Albumin is a protein in the urine that usually enters the urine in minimal quantities. Even a small increase in the level of albumin in the urine in some people may be an early sign of incipient kidney disease, especially in those with diabetes and high blood pressure. In the case of normal kidney function, albumin in the urine should be no more than 3 mg/mmol (or 30 mg/g). If albumin excretion increases even more, then it already speaks of kidney disease. If albumin excretion exceeds 300 mg/g, other proteins are excreted into the urine, and this condition is called proteinuria.

If the kidney is healthy, then albumin does not enter the urine.
In the case of an injured kidney, albumin begins to enter the urine.
If, after receiving the results of the urine analysis, the doctor suspects that there is a kidney disease, then an additional urine analysis is performed for albumin. If albuminuria or proteinuria is detected again within three months, then this indicates chronic kidney disease.

## Additional Examinations

Kidney ultrasound examination:in the diagnosis of chronic kidney disease, it is an examination of the primary choice. Ultrasound examination allows one to assess the shape of the kidneys, their size, location, as well as to determine possible changes in the kidney tissue and/or other abnormalities that may interfere with the normal functioning of the kidneys. Ultrasound examination of the kidneys does not require special training and has no risks for the patient.

If necessary, and if any urological disease is suspected, an ultrasound examination of the urinary tract can be prescribed (as well as a residual urine analysis), and an ultrasound examination of the prostate gland can be prescribed for men and referred to a urologist for a consultation. If necessary, and if a gynecological disease is suspected, a woman is referred for consultation to a gynecologist.

## What You Need To Know About The Examination With a Contrast Agent, If You Have Chronic Kidney Disease

Diagnostic examinations such as magnetic resonance imaging, computed tomography, and angiography are used to diagnose and treat various diseases and injuries. In many cases, intravenous and intra-arterial contrast agents (containing iodine or gadolinium) are used, which makes it possible to see the organs or blood vessels under study.

## What Is Particularly Important To Do Before The Survey Pole To Gain In Contrast Substance?

If you are scheduled for an examination with a contrast agent, then you need to determine your GFR.

Together with your doctor, you can discuss and evaluate the benefits or harm to your health. If the survey is still necessary, follow the following preparation rules:

- The day before the survey and the day after the survey, drink plenty of fluids (water, tea, etc.). If you are on treatment in a hospital, then you will be injected with the necessary amount of fluid through a vein by infusion. When staying in hospital treatment after examination with a contrast agent (within 48-96 hours), it is usually prescribed to determine the level of creatinine in the blood to assess renal function. In the outpatient examination with a contrast agent, your family doctor will be able to evaluate your kidney function.

- Discuss with your doctor the questions about which medications should not be taken before the examination with a contrast agent. Some drugs (antibiotics, drugs against high blood pressure, etc.) along with contrasting substances begin to act as a poison. The day before and the day after the examination, in no case should you take metformin - a cure for diabetes.
- Between the two examinations with a contrast agent, at the first opportunity, sufficient time should be left for the contrast agent that was used during the first examination to leave the body. It is important to exclude repeated examinations with a large amount of contrast material.

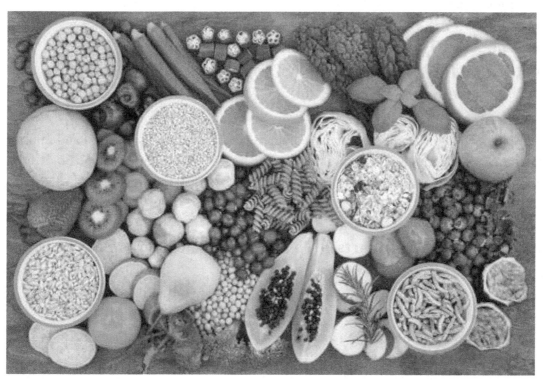

## Treatment Options

The possibilities of treating chronic kidney disease depend on the stage of the severity of the kidney disease, associated diseases and other health problems.

No cure is present for prolonged kidney disease. But some therapies can help in controlling the signs and symptoms, slow down the disease progression, and lessen the danger of complications.

Patients with prolonged kidney disease normally need to take larger doses of medications.

## Treatments include:

- ➢ Anemia treatment. Hemoglobin is an element of the red blood cells that distribute vital oxygen around the body. Shortage of hemoglobin in the body is a sign of anemia. Some kidney disease patients who suffer anemia will need blood transfusions. Usually, a patient with kidney disease will have to replace lost oxygen with an iron supplement, either in daily use of tablets or occasional injections.
- ➢ Phosphate balance. People who suffer from kidney disease may not entirely remove phosphate from their body properly. Therefore, it is recommended that they slow down on their nutritional phosphate intake. By extension, they must reduce the consumption level of dairy products, eggs, fish, and red meat.
- ➢ High blood pressure. HBP is usually associated with patients with chronic kidney disease. In order to protect the kidney, it is necessary to bring the blood pressure down, and consequently, scale down the advancement of the disease.
- ➢ Skin itching. If the patient suffers from skin itching, antihistamines such as chlorpheniramine may be used to reduce the symptoms of itching.
- ➢ Anti-sickness medications. Patients that have kidney problems may find out that they feel sick (nausea) as a result of toxins developing in the body. Medications such as cyclizing or metoclopramide may give them some relief.
- ➢ Nonsteroidal Anti-Inflammatory Drugs (NSAIDs). NSAIDs like ibuprofen or aspirin should not be taken unless prescribed by the physician.
- ➢ End-stage treatment. This happens when the kidney's functionality is between 10-15 percent of standard capacity. Measures listed so far (diet, medications, and treatments) cannot work anymore. End-stage kidney disease patients cannot contain the waste and fluid discharging process. The patient requires an immediate kidney transplant to be alive or at least, regular dialysis to discharge the excess waste and fluid accumulation. Most physicians will probably suspend the need for dialysis or kidney transplant for as long as necessary because of the risk of likely complications associated with transplant and dialysis
- ➢ Kidney dialysis. This is the process of removing waste products and too much fluid from the blood when the kidney fails to function properly. Dialysis has some underlying risks such as infections.

**Dialysis Has Two Main Types And Each Type Has Sub-Types. The Two Main Types Are:**

- Hemodialysis:Here, blood is pumped out of the body and passes through a dialyzer, which serves as the kidney. The patient goes through this about three times a week and one session is about three hours.
- Peritoneal dialysis:A catheter is implanted into the abdomen with which the blood filtration occurs in the patient's own abdomen.
- ➤ **Kidney transplant.** This is the process of swapping the damaged kidney with another if the patient has no other conditions apart from the kidney. A surgical operation is done to effect this change. Both kidney donor and the recipient invariably should have their blood type, cell-surface proteins, and antibodies similar in order to reduce the risk of rejection of the transplanted kidney.

To make the search for a donor short, siblings and close relatives of the kidney patient are the best bet, and if not possible, a search will move to a cadaver donor (dead person).

- ➤ **Vitamin D.** Patients with kidney disease naturally do have a low level of vitamin D. Healthy bones are a result of vitamin D and can be obtained from the sun and food that must be triggered by the kidneys before they are available to the body.
- ➤ **Fluid retention.** People that have chronic disease need to restrict their fluid intake and if the kidney is working properly, the patient risks accumulating a large quantity of liquid.
- ➤ **Diet.** Regulating your diet is important for your treatment of kidney disease to be effective. Reducing the amount of protein in the diet can slow down the progression of the disease.
- ➤ The proper diet may also help in reducing the symptoms of nausea. You must also regulate salt intake as it is associated with hypertension. Potassium and phosphorus consumption may need to be restricted if consumed over a long time.

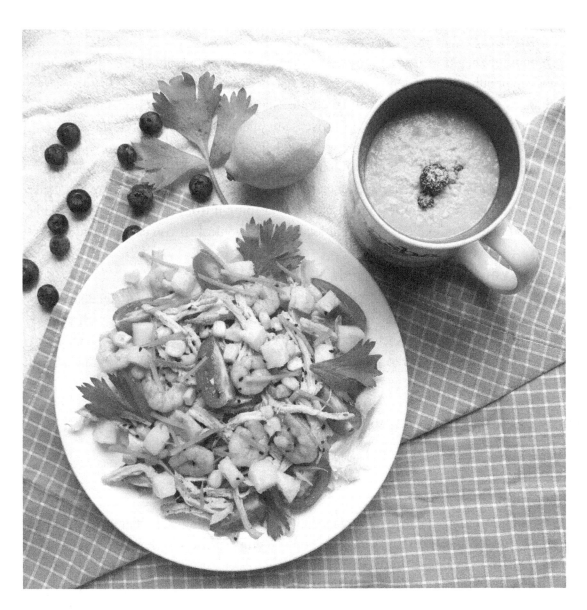

## Slowing Kidney Disease

Now that you know what CKD is, let's look at how to slow the progress. This information will give you specific steps to do to develop a healthier lifestyle and diet. Be open-minded and take it one step at a time. Having a positive attitude is important and the way you embrace the steps will determine how you manage your kidney disease. With some determination and willpower from you, you will soon be in charge of your destiny and health.

## 1. Commit

You might begin feeling a bit overwhelmed when you think about this disease. Take a few deep breaths. Everything is going to be fine because you've got this. Just like any life changes, creating new habits will take time. Start preparing yourself mentally by telling yourself that you can control this disease by managing your lifestyle and diet.

Be determined to change your lifestyle and habits. Your commitment to yourself and your motivation to follow through will help you manage your kidney disease. Keep in mind that the earlier this disease gets detected, the better you can treat it. There is a goal for your treatment:slowing down the disease and keeping it from getting any worse. This is one good thing about kidney disease:it lets you take control so you can manage it.

## 2. Know Your Nutritional Needs

There isn't one diet plan that will be right for everybody who has kidney disease. What you are able to eat is going to change with time. It all depends on how well your kidneys function and factors such as being a diabetic. If you can work closely with your health team and constantly learning, you will be able to make healthy choices that will fit your needs. You can manage your disease and be successful.

## Here Are Some Basic Guidelines That Are Useful For Anyone Who Has Chronic Kidney Disease:

- **Protein**

Protein is present in animal and plant foods. It is a macronutrient that is needed for a healthy body. Too much isn't good for the body. As the function of the kidney's decline, the body doesn't have the ability to get rid of the waste that gets produced when protein gets broken down and it begins to build up in the blood. The correct amount of protein depends on what stage your kidney disease is in, your body size, appetite, levels of albumin, and other factors. A dietitian could help you figure out your daily limits of protein intake. You need to eat 37 to 41 grams of protein daily.

- **Fats**

When you are going through times where you have to restrict what you eat, it is good to know that being able to eat healthy fats is another macronutrient that you need to include daily. Eating healthy fats makes sure you are getting all the essential fatty acids that can help your body in many ways. Polyunsaturated and monounsaturated fats are both unsaturated fats but they are healthy fats because of their benefits to the heart like decreasing LDL, increasing HDL, and lowering the total cholesterol levels. The correct types of fat might decrease inflammation within the body and will protect your kidney from more damage. You should try to include small amounts of these fats into your daily diet.

- **Carbohydrates**

Carbs are another macronutrient that the body needs. This is what the body uses for energy. They also give the body many minerals, fiber, and vitamins that help protect the body. The body needs 130 grams of carbs daily for normal function.

- **Sodium**

Consuming too much sodium makes you thirsty. This can cause increased blood pressure and swelling. Having high blood pressure could cause even more damage to the kidneys that are already unhealthy. Consuming less sodium will lower blood pressure and could slow down chronic kidney disease. The normal recommendation for anyone who has CKD is to keep their sodium intake around 2,000 mg daily. To have the best success is remembering that eating fresh is the best.

- **Potassium**

Potassium can be found in many beverages and foods. It has an important role. It regulates the heartbeat and keeps muscles functioning. People who have kidneys that aren't healthy will need to limit their intake of foods that will increase potassium in the blood. It might increase to dangerous levels. Eating a diet that restricts your level of potassium means eating around 2,000 milligrams each day. Consult your doctor to know the appropriate potassium levels based on your individual needs and blood work.

In order to lessen the buildup of potassium, you have to know what foods are low and high in potassium. This way you know what foods to be careful around.

- **Phosphorus**

Kidneys that are healthy can help the body regulate phosphorus. When you have CKD, your kidneys can't remove excess phosphorus or get rid of it. This results in high levels of phosphorus in the blood and causes the body to pull calcium from bones. This, in turn, will lead the brittle and weak bones. Having elevated levels of calcium and phosphorus could lead to dangerous mineral deposits in the soft tissues of the body. This is called calciphylaxis.

Phosphorus can be found naturally in plant and animal proteins and larger levels are present in processed foods. By choosing foods that are low in phosphorus will keep the phosphorus levels in your body safe. The main rule to keep from eating unwanted phosphorus goes back to "fresh is the best" concept. Basically, stay away from all processed foods. Normal phosphorus intake for anyone who has CKD needs to be around 800 to 1,000 milligrams daily.

- ## Supplements and Vitamins

Instead of relying on supplements, you need to follow a balanced diet. This is the best way to get the number of vitamins your body needs each day. Because of the restrictive CKD diet, it can be hard to get the necessary nutrients and vitamins you need. Anyone who has CKD will have greater needs for vitamins that are water-soluble. Certain renal supplements are needed to get the needed extra water-soluble vitamins. Renal vitamins could be small doses of vitamin C, biotin, pantothenic acid, niacin, folic acid, Vitamins B12, B6, B2, and B1.

The kidney converts inactive vitamin D to an active vitamin D so our bodies can use it. With CKD, kidneys lose the ability to do this. Your health care provider could check your parathyroid hormone, phosphorus, and calcium levels to figure out if you need to take any supplements of active vitamin D. This type of vitamin D requires a prescription.

If your doctor hasn't prescribed a supplement, don't hesitate to ask them if you would benefit from one. To help keep you healthy, only use supplements that have been approved by your dietitian or doctor.

- ## Fluids

A main function for the kidneys is regulating the balance of fluids in the body. For many individuals who have CKD, you don't have to restrict your fluid intake if your output is normal. An increase in the disease contributes to a decline in output and an increase in retention. If this happens, restricting fluids will become necessary. You have to pay attention to how much fluid you are releasing. Let your health care team know if your output is declining. They will be able to tell you how much fluid you should limit on a daily basis to keep healthy fluid levels to prevent an overload of fluid in the body along with other complications that are associated with extra fluid buildups like congestive heart failure, pulmonary edema, and high blood pressure.

## 3. Understand Your Calorie Requirements

Each person's calorie requirements will be different and it doesn't matter if they do or don't have CKD. If they do have CKD, picking the correct foods and eating the right amount of calories will help your body. Calories give us the energy to function daily. They can help to slow the progression of kidney disease, keep a healthy weight, avoid losing muscle mass, prevent infections. Eating too many calories could cause weight gain, and that can put more of a burden on your kidneys. It is important that you get the correct amount of calories. The amount of calories for a person with CKD is about 60 to 70 calories per pound of body weight. If you weigh about 150 pounds, you need to consume around 2,000 calories per day.

## 4. Read Food Labels

It takes time to learn the renal diet and make it a part of your life. Lucky for you, all packaged foods come with nutrition labels along with an ingredient list. You need to read these labels so you can choose the right foods for your nutrition needs.

The major ingredients to check on labels are potassium, phosphorus, sodium, and fat. Food manufacturers should list the sodium and fat content of the food as required by law. They aren't required to list potassium or phosphorus. It is important to find this information in other places like the internet or books.

## 5. Portion Control

When you have kidney disease, controlling your portions is important. This doesn't mean you have to starve yourself. It doesn't matter what stage of CKD you are in but eating moderately is important when preserving your kidney health. The biggest part is making sure you don't feel deprived. You can enjoy many different foods as long as they are kidney-friendly and don't overeat. When you cut back on foods that could harm your health and you are careful about what you eat, you are learning portion control. Make a habit of limiting specific foods and eating in moderation when following a kidney diet. It just takes having an informed game plan, resolve, and time.

Picking the correct foods is critical to your kidneys. They are counting on you to give them the correct nutrients so they can function their best. This include minerals, vitamins, fats, carbohydrates, and protein. Too much of any one could harm your body and make your kidneys work harder to get rid of the toxins.

# Chapter 2: The Renal Diet Explained

Bad eating habits can have adverse effects on your health. If you want to avoid kidney diseases, you must manage a balanced diet and stay at a healthy weight. Your diet is supposed to contain low levels of fat and salt to control blood pressure. A diabetic person must control his/her blood sugar by choosing the right food and beverages. Control diabetes and high blood pressure to prevent the worse condition of kidney disease. Only a kidney-friendly diet can help you in the protection of kidneys from more damage. By choosing a kidney-friendly diet, you can limit particular foods to avoid the build-up of minerals in your body.

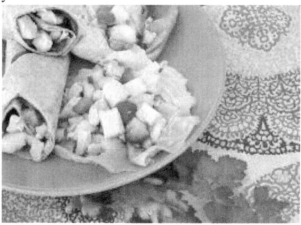

## Understand Your Nutrient Needs

When following a renal diet, certain nutrients are very important as they can actually make worse or improve chronic kidney disorder. Some of the vital ones include:

### Potassium.

Potassium is a naturally occurring mineral found in nearly all foods, in varying amounts. Our bodies need an amount of potassium to help with muscle activity as well as electrolyte balance and regulation of blood pressure. However, if potassium is in excess within the system and the kidneys can't expel it (due to renal disease), fluid retention and muscle spasms can occur.

## Phosphorus.

Phosphorus is a trace mineral found in a wide range of foods and especially dairy, meat, and eggs. It acts synergistic-ally with calcium as well as Vitamin D to promote bone health. However, when there is damage in the kidneys, excess amounts of the mineral cannot be taken out and this can cause bone weakness.

## Calories.

When being on a renal diet, it is important to give yourself the right amount of calories to fuel your system. The exact amount of calories you should consume daily depends on your age, gender, general health status and stage of renal disease. In most cases though, there are no strict limitations in the calorie intake, as long as you take them from proper sources that are low in sodium, potassium, and phosphorus. In general, doctors recommend a daily limit between 1800-2100 calories per day to keep weight within the normal range.

## Protein.

Protein is an essential nutrient that our systems need to develop and generate new connective tissue e.g. muscles, even during injuries. Protein also helps stop bleeding and supports the immune system fight infections. A healthy adult with no kidney disease would normally need 40-65 grams of protein per day.

However, in renal diet, protein consumption is a tricky subject as too much or too little can cause problems. Protein, when being metabolized by our systems also creates waste which is typically processed by the kidneys. But when kidneys are damaged or under performing, as in the case of kidney disease that waste will stay in the system. This is why patients in more advanced CKD stages are advised to limit their protein consumption as well.

## Fats.

Fats and particularly good fats are needed by our systems as a fuel source and for other metabolic cell functions. A diet rich in bad and trans or saturated fats though can greatly raise the odds of developing heart problems, which often occur with the renal disease. This is why most physicians advise their renal patients to follow a diet that contains a decent amount of good fats and a very low amount of trans (processed) or saturated fat.

## Sodium.

Sodium is an essential mineral that our bodies need to regulate fluid and electrolyte balance. It also plays a role in normal cell division in the muscles and nervous system. However, in kidney disease, sodium can quickly spike at higher than normal levels and the kidneys will be unable to expel it causing fluid accumulation as a side-effect. Those who also suffer from heart problems as well should limit its consumption as it may raise blood pressure.

## Carbohydrates.

Carbs act as a major and quick fuel source for the body's cells. When we consume carbs, our systems turn them into glucose and then into energy for "feeding" our body cells. Carbs are generally not restricted in the renal diet but some types of carbs contain dietary fiber as well, which helps regulate normal colon function and protect blood vessels from damage.

## Dietary Fiber.

Fiber is an important element in our system that cannot be properly digested but plays a key role in the regulation of our bowel movements and blood cell protection. The fiber in the renal diet is generally encouraged as it helps loosen up the stools, relieve constipation and bloating and protect from colon damage. However, many patients don't get enough amounts of dietary fiber per day as many of them are high in potassium or phosphorus. Fortunately, there are some good dietary fiber sources for CKD patients that have lower amounts of these minerals compared to others.

## Vitamins/Minerals.

Our systems, according to medical research, need at least 13 vitamins and minerals to keep our cells fully active and healthy. Patients with renal disease though are more likely to be depleted by water-soluble vitamins like B-complex and Vitamin C, as a result, or limited fluid consumption. Therefore, supplementation with these vitamins along with a renal diet program should help cover any possible vitamin deficiencies. Supplementation of fat-soluble vitamins like vitamins A, K, and E may be avoided as they can quickly build up in the system and turn toxic.

## Fluids.

When you are in an advanced stage of renal disease, fluid can quickly build-up and lead to problems. While it is important to keep your system well hydrated, you should avoid minerals like potassium and sodium which can trigger further fluid build-up and cause a host of other symptoms.

# Nutrients You Need To Avoid

Salt or sodium is known for being one of the most important ingredients that the renal diet prohibits its use. This ingredient, although simple, can badly and strongly affect your body and especially the kidneys. Any excess of sodium can't be easily filtered because of the failing condition of the kidneys. A large build-up of sodium can cause catastrophic results on your body. Potassium and Phosphorus are also prohibited for kidney patients depending on the stage of kidney disease.

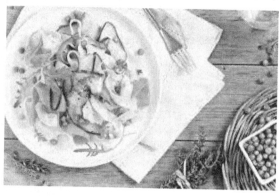

# Adopting a New Lifestyle To Minimize Your Kidney Problems

When you are recovering from acute renal failure or when you are on a renal failure diet, then your doctor or dietician would recommend a particular diet that would help you in limiting the stress on your kidneys. Your dietician would analyze and depending upon your current situation would suggest a diet that would reduce the pressure on your kidneys. Here are certain lifestyle changes that would help you in the recovery process and also help you to have healthy kidneys.

You should opt for foods that have a low level of potassium or no potassium at all. Foods rich in potassium include bananas, spinach, tomatoes, oranges and even potatoes. You can instead consume foods that have a low level of potassium in them like apples, cabbage, grapes, strawberries and green beans as well. You should avoid products that have added salt in them. You should cut down on the amount of sodium that you consume on a daily basis and this can be done by simply avoiding packed and canned foods, even frozen foods, you should also avoid processed meats as well as cheeses. Phosphorus is generally found in dairy products like milk, cheese and butter. It is also present in beans and nuts. You will need to reduce the amount of phosphorus that you consume because this weakens your bones and also cause skin irritation. Once your kidneys start recovering, your diet would change but that doesn't mean that you should stop eating healthy foods.

You should reduce or eliminate emotional stress. Quit smoking, alcohol consumption or any drugs not prescribed by a doctor.

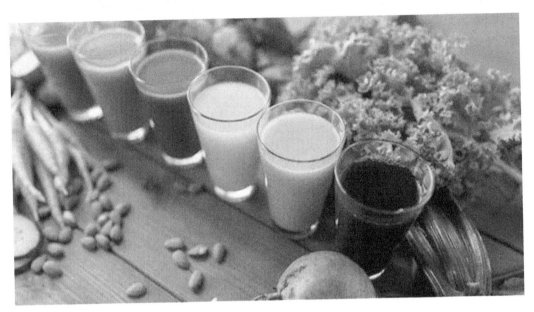

# Managing Your Renal Diet When You Are Diabetic

## What is diabetes?

It is a chronic disease where the patient has higher levels of blood sugar beyond the normal one. Also, there are metabolic disorders of carbohydrates, fats, and proteins. Normal in a healthy person, the pancreas secretes insulin in an amount sufficient to balance the blood sugar level. In the case of diabetes, insulin secretion from the pancreas is disturbed, and insulin is released too little, or its secretion stops. Therefore, blood sugar levels begin to rise. This condition begins to disrupt the work of muscles and many other organs, including the kidneys, heart, blood vessels, nerves, and eyes.

## Type I Diabetes

It usually begins in childhood and occurs if the body cannot produce insulin in the right amount. Insulin treatment is always used to keep blood sugar levels under control.

## Type II diabetes.

Can form slowly and at first without symptoms. The causes of type II diabetes are predominantly heredity (the presence of a disease in close relatives), overweight, metabolic syndrome (elevated pressure, obesity in the lumbar region, elevated blood pressure), and diabetes of pregnant women. If a person has type II diabetes, his body still produces insulin, but its level is very low, or it cannot be used in the right way.

For type II diabetes, the sugar level can sometimes be kept under control with proper nutrition/diet or physical activity, but usually, pills and/or insulin are still needed.

To prevent kidney damage and to slow the progression of the disease, it is essential to keep blood sugar levels under control.

Blood level in the blood can be measured independently using a glucometer. So you can measure your blood sugar level yourself and keep it at the correct level. Ask for advice and more information from your family doctor/nurse, endocrinologist, or nurse who specializes in diabetes.

# Shopping List for Week 1 And 2

Almonds
Apples
Arugula
Asparagus
Basil
Bass fillets
Beef steak
Berries - Blueberries, blackberries, strawberries
Carrots
Cauliflower
Chicken breasts
Chives
Cod
Cucumbers
Cumin
Eggs
Flour

Garlic cloves
Ginger
Green beans
Lemon
Lettuce
Olive oil
Onions
Pears
Pineapples
Red peppers
Salmon
Shrimp
Sirloin roast
Squash
Tofu
Tuna
Turkey breasts

# Week 1 Meal Plan

| Day | Breakfast | Lunch | Dinner | Snack/Dessert/Salad |
|---|---|---|---|---|
| 1 | Poached Asparagus and Egg | Shrimp Paella | Grilled Spiced Turkey | Mock Pancakes |
| 2 | Apple Turnover | Salmon & Pesto Salad | Ginger & Bean Sprout Steak Stir-Fry | Breakfast Cheesecake |
| 3 | Egg Drop Soup | Roast Beef | Baked Fennel & Garlic Sea Bass | Mock Cream Cheese Pancake |
| 4 | Summer Squash and Apple Soup | Lemon, Garlic & Cilantro Tuna And Rice | Carrot & Ginger Chicken Noodles | Pear & Brie Salad |
| 5 | Roasted Pepper Soup | Thai Tofu Broth | Shrimp Paella | Caesar Salad |
| 6 | Power-Boosting Smoothie | Herby Chicken Stew | Lemon & Herb Chicken Wraps | Cucumber Salad |
| 7 | Distinctive Pineapple Smoothie | Chili Tofu Noodles | Cod & Green Bean Risotto | Thai Cucumber Salad |

# Week 2 Meal Plan

| Day | Breakfast | Lunch | Dinner | Snack/Dessert/Salad |
|---|---|---|---|---|
| 1 | Strengthening Smoothie Bowl | Baked Fennel & Garlic Sea Bass | Beef Brochetes | Raspberry Muffins |
| 2 | Brilliant Berry Smoothie | Curried Cauliflower | Ginger & Bean Sprout Steak Stir-Fry | Kidney-friendly Unsalted Pretzels |
| 3 | Poached Asparagus and Egg | Cod & Green Bean Risotto | Carrot & Ginger Chicken Noodles | Vanilla Custard |
| 4 | Summer Squash and Apple Soup | Salmon & Pesto Salad | Chinese Tempeh Stir Fry | Almond Cookies |
| 5 | Apple Turnover | Grilled Spiced Turkey | Delicious Vegetarian Lasagne | Cucumber Salad |
| 6 | Distinctive Pineapple Smoothie | Lemon & Herb Chicken Wraps | Lemon, Garlic & Cilantro Tuna And Rice | Mock Cream Cheese Pancake |
| 7 | Egg Drop Soup | Chinese Tempeh Stir Fry | Roast Beef | Raspberry Muffins |

# Shopping List for Week 3 And 4

Almond milk
Apples
Asparagus
Bananas
Basil
Beef steak
Berries - raspberries, blueberries, cranberries, strawberries
Bone/chuck roast
Carrots

Cauliflowers
Chives
Cinnamon
Collard greens
Dates
Eggs
Flour
Garlic cloves
Ginger
Grapes
Green beans

Green, black, red and yellow peppers
Haddock fillets
Halibut fillet
Lean lamb
Lemons
Lime
Mayonnaise
Olive oil
Onions
Peaches

Red pepper flakes  Shallots  White rice
Pineapples  Tempeh  Yellow and red bell
Pork and Bacon  Tofu  peppers
Red chili  Trout  Zucchinis
Red potatoes  Tuna

# Week 3 Meal Plan

| Day | Breakfast | Lunch | Dinner | Snack/Dessert/Salad |
|---|---|---|---|---|
| 1 | Assorted Fresh Fruit Juice (Beverage) | Parsley Root Veg Stew | Beef Pot Roast | Eggs Creamy Melt |
| 2 | Raspberry and Pineapple Smoothie (Dairy-Free) | Mixed Pepper Stuffed River Trout | Meat Loaf | Mashed Cauliflowers |
| 3 | Mexican Frittata | Mixed Pepper Paella | Pork Loins with Leeks | Banana Cookies |
| 4 | Olive Oil and Sesame Asparagus | Chinese Beef Wraps | Haddock & Buttered Leeks | Baked Cinnamon over Apple Raisins |
| 5 | Pineapple Juice | Country Fried Steak | Spiced Lamb Burgers | Red Potato Salad |
| 6 | Blueberry Burst | Cauliflower Rice & Runny Eggs | Homemade Tuna Nicoise | Broccoli-Cauliflower Salad |
| 7 | Peach Iced-Tea | Thai Spiced Halibut | Pork Loins with Leeks | Macaroni Salad |

# Week 4 Meal Plan

| Day | Breakfast | Lunch | Dinner | Snack/Dessert/Salad |
|---|---|---|---|---|
| 1 | Lemon Boost | Monk-Fish Curry | Country Fried Steak | Green Bean and Potato Salad |
| 2 | Mexican Frittata | Minted Zucchini Noodles | Meat Loaf | Chocolate Chip Cookies |
| 3 | Assorted Fresh Fruit Juice (Beverage) | Mini Burgers | Mixed Pepper Stuffed River Trout | Fruit Compote |
| 4 | Olive Oil and Sesame Asparagus | Homemade Tuna Nicoise | Beef Pot Roast | Puffed Cereal Bars |
| 5 | Blueberry Burst | Chili Tempeh & Scallions | Monk-Fish Curry | Strawberry Ice-cream |
| 6 | Pineapple Juice | Haddock & Buttered Leeks | Chinese Beef Wraps | Mashed Cauliflowers |
| 7 | Raspberry and Pineapple Smoothie (Dairy-Free) | Spiced Lamb Burgers | Thai Spiced Halibut | Broccoli-Cauliflower Salad |

# Chapter 3: Tips and FAQs

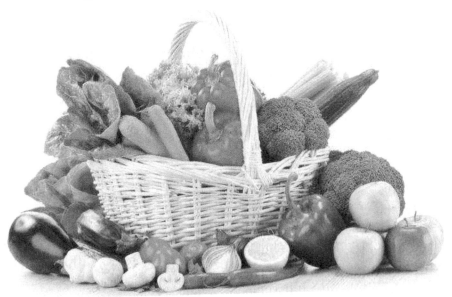

## Tips On Controlling Your Phosphorus

Phosphorus is a well-known mineral that the body can get rid of through the urine thanks to the help of healthy kidneys. However, if kidneys malfunction, phosphorus starts building up in the blood vessels and this may result in many serious health problems. The inability of kidneys to remove extra phosphorus from the body can cause several pains like, heart calcification, joint pain and leads to easily broken bones.

Phosphorus has always been related to the health of the bone and together with calcium bones are indispensable for maintaining strong bones. And in order to keep the level of phosphorus balanced in your body, you should carefully watch the foods you eat like meats, poultry, fish, beans, nuts and dairy products. Phosphorus is more likely to be found in animal foods and plant foods, yet our body absorbs the phosphorus we get from animal foods more than from plant foods.

The phosphorus that is added to certain foods is not as healthy as we can imagine because it comes in the form of preservatives and additives and it can be found in fast and junk foods. We might not know that our body totally absorbs the phosphorus that we get from food additives. Hence, avoiding additives is the best way we can use to lower the intake of phosphorus additives. You should always check the facts on the label of each food you buy and search for the "Phos" to be able to know which contains more phosphorous.

In order to maintain a balanced level of phosphorous and to keep it under control; here is what you should do:

Limit the consumption of foods like poultry, meats, fish and dairy

- Limit the intake of certain dairy products like yogurt and cheese; you should not exceed 4 oz per serving
- Avoid black beans, lima beans, red beans, garbanzo beans, white beans and black-eyed peas.
- Avoid unrefined, whole and dark grains.
- Stay away from refrigerator dough
- Avoid dried fruits and vegetables
- Avoid chocolate
- Avoid sodas that are dark-colored
- Make sure to take your phosphate binders with your snacks and meals.
- The renal diet limits the intake of phosphorus to 1000mg per day

# Tips on Controlling your Protein

Protein makes an essential element of our growth and it plays an important role in maintaining our body mass. Besides, proteins can help us fight any infection that can threaten our bodies. And while proteins are very important for our health, excessive consumption may lead to undesirable and even threatening results. In fact, eating more than your body needs can hasten the deterioration of your kidneys.

Therefore, maintaining a moderate and balanced intake of proteins can keep your body healthy and it can prevent kidney failure. Furthermore, when your kidneys are not able to function very well; they start leaking protein into your urine and this can lead to many unpleasant side effects like a change in taste, loss of appetite, nausea and even fatigue.

In a few words, protein is very important for the growth and the maintenance of our health and it is substantial in healing wounds, fighting all infections and providing our body with the energy it needs. Nevertheless, it's substantial to keep the level of proteins in our bodies balanced.

To make sure that our kidneys are not stressed by the proteins we eat, we should make sure to consume high-quality proteins. And we should make sure that we eat about 7 to 8 oz. of protein per day. 1 Egg equals 1 oz. of protein.

Pork, beef, turkey, veal; chicken and eggs have high amounts of protein.

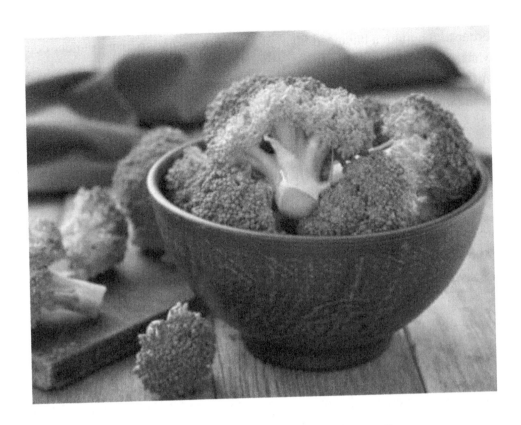

# Tips on Controlling Your Fluid Intake

When your kidneys function properly, they are able to get rid of the fluids that enter our body. However, when our kidneys are not working properly and, our body might not be able to get rid of the fluids as it used to. The buildup of fluids in our body can lead to swelling, high blood pressure and even shortness of breath.

Therefore, we should limit our intake of fluids and keep it under control so that we can avoid dialysis at a certain step. There are lots of foods high in water like ice cream, sauces, rice pudding, gravy and custard. You should cut down on some food packed with water and avoid some other foods as well. Moreover, people who suffer from kidney diseases and who consume high levels of fluids may experience pressure on the heart and the lungs.

**And Here Are Some Tips With Which You Can Restrict The Intake Of Fluids:**

1.  Use 1 cup or glass in order to divide your fluid intake per day. You can also write a record of your fluid intake.
2.  Always avoid any type of salty food and never add extra salt to your meals.
3.  Avoid processed meats, fast foods and canned foods
4.  You can add lemon juice to the water you want to drink instead

5. You can rinse your mouth with a mouthwash from time to time
6. Avoid overheating
7. Maintain your blood sugar at a balanced level

# Eating out

You can still enjoy your favorite restaurant or cuisines! Look out for small or half portions and ask your server for your foods to be cooked without extra salts, butter or sauces. Avoid fried foods. Instead, embrace poached or grilled food.

If you know you are going out to eat, plan ahead. Look at the restaurant's menu beforehand and decide what you will order to avoid anxiety or stress on the night! Be sure to take your phosphorus binders, if they have been prescribed to you. Take them with your meal instead of waiting until you get home.

# FAQs

**Q:How Can i Figure Out If a Food Label Or Recipe Is Low In Potassium And What Is The Maximum Daily Limit?**

**A:**When following a renal diet, you ideally want to make sure that potassium levels are below 250mg/per serving or up to 7% of the food's total nutritional value. If the food/recipe indicates less than 100 mg of potassium per serving, this means that it's very low in potassium. However, a moderate rate of up to 250 mg per serving is fine, as long as you don't consume any other foods throughout the day with moderate or high potassium levels e.g. between 250-400 mg/serving.

**Q:Can One Lose Weight During a Renal Diet?**

**A:**If you wish to lose extra weight for health or fitness reasons, you can follow a renal diet plan that is preferably high in fats and fiber foods e.g. forest fruits, cabbage, etc. You still want to make sure that your daily calorie intake does not exceed 2000 calories and any foods that you choose are low in sodium and potassium to keep bloating and fluid build-up under control. The exact amount of calories that you need to take though, depends on your age, gender, health status and the weight goal that you wish to achieve. If you wish to lose weight as well with your renal diet plan, it's better to discuss the matter with an expert dietician or nutritionist.

**Q:Does My Ckd Stage Count When Following a Renal Diet?**

**A:**Absolutely! In earlier stages (up to the third stage), it is fine to consume low to moderate amounts of sodium, potassium, and phosphorus while your fluid intake should be up to 2.5 liters per day. However, when you are in a more advanced stage of renal damage, you have to limit all the above minerals and fluids further e.g. drink up to 2 liters of fluids per day or only up to 150 mg of potassium per meal (instead of 250mg). Your doctor or dietician will give you additional guidelines on the exact amounts of each that you need to take daily, based on your current stage of renal disease.

**Q:Is It OK To Take Caffeine In a Renal Diet?**

**A:**In most cases and especially during the first three stages of CKD, a caffeine-based drink is perfectly fine. You may drink up to 2 cups of coffee or caffeine tea per day without any worries. However, be careful as any extras that you add to your coffee will not only increase calories, they may raise potassium levels as well. Such toppings are whipping cream, caramel syrups, chocolate, etc. Pure coffee or black tea with water and a bit of almond or soy milk isn't an issue but anything "fortified" should be avoided.

**Q:Can i Take Over The Counter Medication When On a Renal Diet?**

**A:**Unfortunately, the vast majority of over the counter medication/painkillers like aspirin and ibuprofen are not indicated for CKD patients. Any drug that belongs in the NSAID (nonsteroidal anti-inflammatory drugs) category should be avoided. According to some studies, NSAIDs can worsen CKD. Some other types of medication are also not indicated for renal patients. If you are currently taking any other medication, it would be wise to consult your doctor to find out whether they are OK for kidney function or not.

# Chapter 4: The Delicious Recipes

It is essential to enjoy a sumptuous but healthy breakfast, quick lunch, and dinner. The breakfast recipes outlined in this section will leap-start your day and keep you going all through the day! You will enjoy the quick lunch recipes. Dinner is a very important time that you will gather together as a family and enjoy the best food. Try out the following recipes.

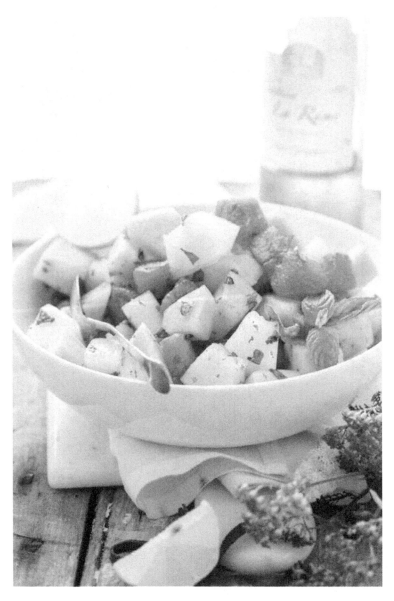

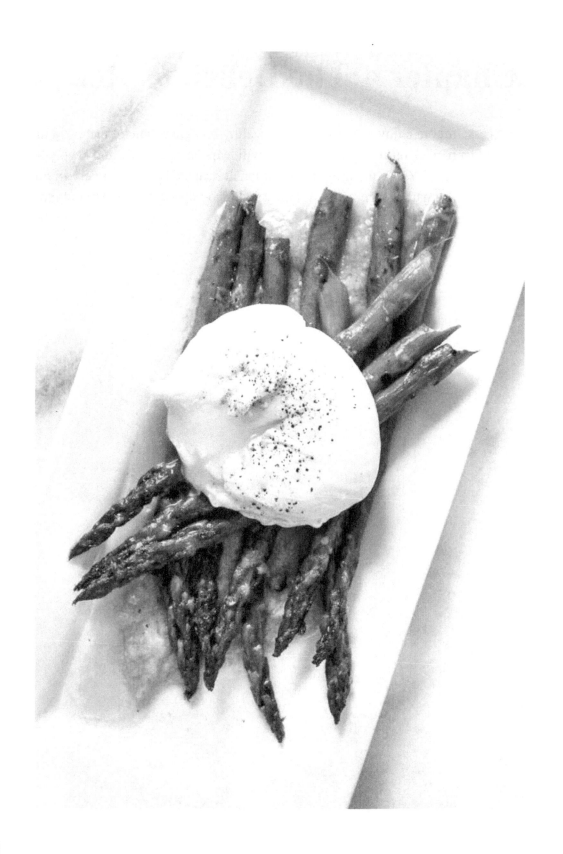

# Breakfast

## Poached Asparagus and Egg

Prep time:3 minutes, Cook time:15 minutes, Servings:1

**Ingredients:**

- 1 egg
- 4 spears asparagus
- Water

**Preparation:**

1. Half-fill a deep saucepan with water set over high heat. Let the water come to a boil.
2. Dip asparagus spears in water. Cook until they turn a shade brighter, about 3 minutes. Remove from saucepan and drain on paper towels. Keep warm. Lightly season prior to serving.
3. Using a slotted spoon, gently lower egg into boiling water. Cook for only 4 minutes. Remove from pan immediately. Place on egg holder.
4. Slice off the top. The egg should still be fluid inside.
5. Place asparagus spears on a small plate and serve egg on the side. Dip asparagus into the egg and eat while warm.

**Nutritional information:**

Calories 178, Carbs 1g, Fat 13g, Protein 7.72g, Potassium (K) 203 mg, Sodium (Na) 71 mg, Phosphorus 124 mg

# Apple Turnover

Prep time: 10 minutes, Cook time:15 minutes, Servings:8

**Ingredients:**

**For the turnovers:**

- ½ tsp. cinnamon powder
- All-purpose flour
- ½ cup unwashed palm sugar
- 1 tbsp. almond flour
- 1 frozen puff pastry
- 4 peeled, cored and diced baking apples.

**For the egg wash:**

- 2 tbsps. Water
- 1 whisked egg white

**Preparation:**

1. To make the filling:combine almond flour, cinnamon powder and palm sugar until these resemble coarse meal. Toss in diced apples until well coated. Set aside.
2. On a lightly floured surface, roll out the puff pastry until ¼ inch thin. Slice into 8 pieces of 4" x 4" squares.
3. Divide the prepared apples into 8 equal portions. Spoon on individual puff pastry squares. Fold in half diagonally. Press edges to seal.
4. Place each filled pastry on a baking tray lined with parchment paper. Make sure there is ample space between pastries.
5. Freeze for at least 20 minutes, or until ready to bake.
6. Preheat oven to 400°F for 10 minutes.
7. Brush frozen pastries with egg wash. Place in the hot oven, and cook for 12 to 15 minutes, or until they turn golden brown all over.
8. Remove baking tray from oven immediately. Cool slightly for easier handling.
9. Place 1 apple turnover on a plate. Serve warm.

**Nutritional information:**

Protein 3.81g, Potassium (K) 151 mg, Sodium (Na) 86 mg, Carbs 35.75g, Calories 285, Fat 14.78g, Phosphorus 43.4mg

# Egg Drop Soup

Prep time: 5 minutes, Cook time:10 minutes , Servings:4

**Ingredients:**

- ¼ cup minced fresh chives
- 4 cups unsalted vegetable stock
- 4 whisked eggs

**Preparation:**

1. Pour unsalted vegetable stock into the oven set over high heat. Bring to a boil. Turn down heat to the lowest heat setting.
2. Pour in the eggs. Stir continuously until ribbons form into the soup.
3. Turn off the heat immediately. The residual heat will cook eggs through.
4. Cool slightly before ladling the desired amount into individual bowls. Garnish with a pinch of parsley, if using. Serve immediately.

**Nutritional information:**

Calories 32, Carbs 0g, Fat 2 g, Protein 5.57g, Potassium (K) 67 mg, Sodium (Na) 63 mg, Phosphorus 36.1mg

# Summer Squash and Apple Soup

Prep time:10 minutes, Cook Time:40 minutes , Servings:4

## Ingredients:

- 1 cup non-dairy milk
- ½ tsp. cumin
- 3 cups unsalted vegetable broth
- 1 ½ tsps. Grated ginger
- 1 tbsp. olive oil
- 1 lb. peeled summer squash
- 2 diced apples
- ¾ tsp. curry powder

## Preparation:

1. Set the oven to 375 °F.
2. Cut out a sheet of aluminum foil that is big enough to wrap the summer squash. Once wrapped, bake for 30 minutes.
3. Remove the wrapped summer squash from the oven and set aside to cool.
4. Once cooled, remove the aluminum foil, remove the seeds, and peel.
5. Dice the summer squash, then place in a food processor. Add non-dairy milk. Blend until smooth. Transfer to a bowl and set aside.
6. Place a soup pot over medium flame and heat through. Once hot, add the olive oil and swirl to coat.
7. Sauté the onion until tender, then add the diced apple, spices, and broth. Bring to a boil. Once boiling, reduce to a simmer and let simmer for about 8 minutes.
8. Turn off the heat and let cool slightly. Once cooled, pour the mixture into the food processor and blend until smooth.
9. Pour the pureed apple mixture back into the pot, then stir in the summer squash mixture. Mix well, then reheat to a simmer over medium flame. Serve.

## Nutritional information:

Calories 240, Protein 2.24g, Potassium (K) 376 mg, Sodium (Na) 429 mg, Fat 8g, Carbs 40g, Phosphorus 0g

# Roasted Pepper Soup

Prep time:10 minutes, Cook Time:30 minutes , Servings:4

## Ingredients:

- 2 cups unsalted vegetable broth
- ½ cup chopped carrots
- 2 large red peppers
- ¼ cup julienned sweet basil
- 2 minced garlic cloves
- ½ cup chopped celery
- 2 tbsps. Olive oil
- ½ cup chopped onion
- ½ cup almond milk

## Preparation:

1. Place the oven into the 375°F.
2. Put onions on a baking sheet. Add the red peppers beside the mixture. Drizzle some of the olive oil over everything and toss well to coat.
3. Roast for 20 minutes, or until peppers are tender and skins are wilted.
4. Chop the roasted red peppers and set aside.
5. Place a pot over medium high flame and heat through. Once hot, add the olive oil and swirl to coat.
6. Place the carrot, celery, and garlic into the pot and sauté until carrot and celery are tender. Add the chopped roasted red peppers. Mix well.
7. Pour in the vegetable broth and almond milk. Increase to high flame and bring to a boil.
8. Once boiling, reduce to a simmer. Simmer, uncovered, for 10 minutes.
9. Turn off the heat and allow to cool slightly.
10. If desired, blend the soup using an immersion blender until the soup has reached a desired level of smoothness. Reheat over medium flame.
11. Add the basil and stir to combine. Serve.

## Nutritional information:

Calories 320, Protein 1.3g, Potassium (K) 249 mg, Sodium (Na) 45 mg Fat 25g, Carbs 20g, Phosphorus 66.33 g

# Assorted Fresh Fruit Juice (Beverage)

Prep time:5 minutes , Cook time:0 minutes , Servings:1

**Ingredients:**

- 1 roughly chopped apple
- ¼ cup halved frozen grapes
- 1 cup ice shavings

**Preparation:**

1. Add all ingredients into the blender.
2. Process until smooth.
3. Pour equal portions into glasses. Serve immediately.

**Nutritional information:**

Calories 112, Protein 1.16g, Potassium (K) 367 mg, Sodium (Na) 3 mg, Fat 0.5g, Carbs 25.8g Phosphorus 17.4mg

# Raspberry and Pineapple Smoothie (Dairy-Free)

Prep time: 5 minutes, Cook time:5 minutes , Servings:4

**Ingredients:**

- ½ cup crushed ice
- 1 chopped small overripe banana piece
- 8 oz. rinsed and drained pineapple tidbits
- ½ cup frozen raspberries

**Preparation:**

1. Except for cashew nuts and stevia, combine remaining ingredients in a deep microwave-safe bowl. Stir.
2. Microwave on the highest setting for 5 to 15 seconds. Keep a watchful eye on this. Stop the cooking process before milk bubbles out of the bowl.
3. Carefully remove the bowl from microwave. Cool slightly for easier handling.
4. Stir in stevia if using. Sprinkle cashew nuts.

**Nutritional information:**

Protein 3.1g, Potassium (K) 749 mg, Sodium (Na) 4 mg, Calories 360, Fat 1g, Carbs 90g, Phosphorus 106.2mg

# Mexican Frittata

Prep time:5 minutes, Cook time:20 minutes Servings:2

## Ingredients:

- 5 large eggs
- ¼ cup chopped green bell pepper
- ¼ cup chopped onions
- ½ cup almond milk

## Preparation:

1. Preheat the oven to 400° F.
2. Using a large bowl, combine almond milk, eggs, onion, and green bell pepper. Whisk until all ingredients are well combined.
3. Transfer the mixture to a baking dish. Bake for 20 minutes. Serve.

## Nutritional information:

Calories 239.5, Protein 16.35g, Potassium (K) 243 mg, Sodium (Na) 216 mg, Carbs 5.3 g, Fat 17.0 g, Phosphorus 94 mg

# Olive Oil and Sesame Asparagus

Prep time:5 minutes, Cook Time:5 minutes , Servings:1

**Ingredients:**

- ½ tbsp. olive oil
- 2 cups sliced asparagus
- ½ cup water
- ½ tsp. sesame seeds
- 1/8 tsp. crushed red pepper flakes

**Preparation:**

1. In a large skillet, bring water to a boil.
2. Add in asparagus. Allow to boil for 2 minutes. Reduce the heat and cook for another 5 minutes. Drain asparagus and place on a plate. Set aside.
3. Meanwhile, heat the olive oil. Tip in asparagus and red pepper flakes. Saute for 3 minutes.
4. Remove from heat. Drizzle in more olive oil and sprinkle sesame seeds before serving.

**Nutritional information:**

Calories 122, Protein 6.19g, Potassium (K) 547 mg, Sodium (Na) 9 mg Fat 7g, Carbs 11g, Phosphorus:37mg

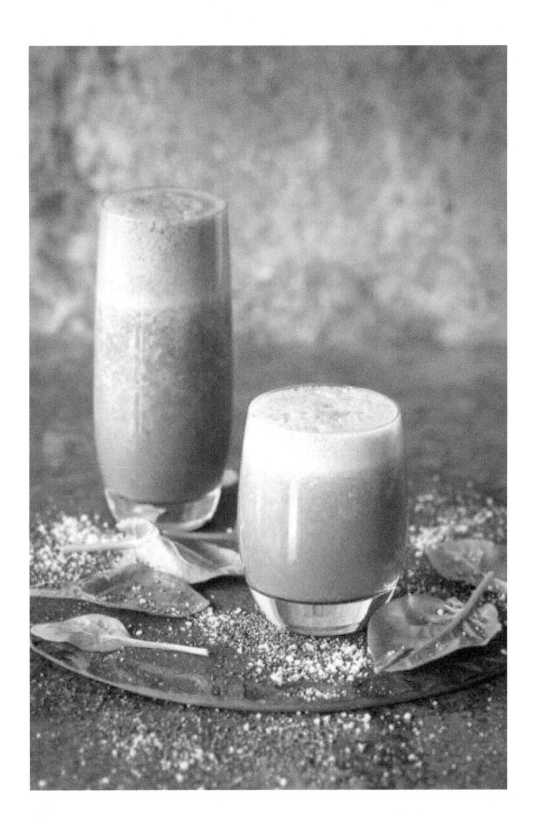

# Smoothies and drinks

## Power-Boosting Smoothie

Prep time:5 minutes, Cook time:, Servings:2

**Ingredients:**

- ½ cup water
- ½ cup non-dairy whipped topping
- 2 scoops whey protein powder
- 1½ cups frozen blueberries

**Directions:**

1. In a high-speed blender, add all ingredients and pulse till smooth.
2. Transfer into 2 serving glass and serve immediately.

**Nutritional information:**

Calories 242, Fat 7g, Carbs 23.8g, Protein 23.2g, Potassium (K) 263mg, Sodium (Na) 63mg, Phosphorous 30 mg

## Distinctive Pineapple Smoothie

Prep time:5 minutes, Cook time:0 minutes, Servings:2

**Ingredients:**

- ¼ cup crushed ice cubes
- 2 scoops vanilla whey protein powder
- 1 cup water
- 1½ cups pineapple

**Preparation:**

1. In a high-speed blender, add all ingredients and pulse till smooth.
2. Transfer into 2 serving glass and serve immediately.

**Nutritional information:**

Calories 117, Fat 2.1g, Carbs 18.2g, Protein 22.7g, Potassium (K) 296mg, Sodium (Na) 81mg, Phosphorous 28 mg

# Strengthening Smoothie Bowl

Prep time:5 minutes, Cook time:4 minutes, Servings:2

**Ingredients:**

- ¼ cup fresh blueberries
- ¼ cup fat-free plain Greek yogurt
- 1/3 cup unsweetened almond milk
- 2 tbsps. whey protein powder
- 2 cups frozen blueberries

**Preparation:**

1. In a blender, add blueberries and pulse for about 1 minute.
2. Add almond milk, yogurt and protein powder and pulse till desired consistency.
3. Transfer the mixture into 2 bowls evenly.
4. Serve with the topping of fresh blueberries.

**Nutritional information:**

Calories 176, Fat 2.1g, Carbs 27g., Protein 15.1g, Potassium (K) 242mg, Sodium (Na) 72mg, Phosphorous 555.3 mg

# Brilliant Berry Smoothie

Prep time:5 minutes, Cook time:0 minutes, Servings:2

**Ingredients:**

- ¼ cup blackberries
- ¼ cup unenriched rice milk.
- ¼ cup sliced strawberries
- ¼ cup blueberries

**Preparation:**

1. Blend in a food processor or smoothie maker and serve over ice if desired.
2. Enjoy!

**Nutritional information:**

Calories:90, Fat 1g, Carbs 18g, Phosphorus 82mg, Potassium (K) 70mg, Sodium (Na) 30mg, Protein:1g

# Pineapple Juice

Prep time:5 minutes, Cook time:0 minutes, Servings:2

**Ingredients:**

- ½ cup canned pineapple
- 1 cup water

**Preparation:**

1. Blend all ingredients and serve over ice.

**Nutritional information:**

Calories 135, Protein 0 g, Carbs 0 g, Fat 0 g, Sodium (Na) 0 mg, Potassium (K) 180 mg, Phosphorus 8 mg

# Blueberry Burst

Prep time:5 minutes, Cook time:0 minutes, Servings:2

**Ingredients:**

- 1 cup chopped collard greens
- 1 cup unsweetened rice milk
- 1 tbsp. almond butter
- 1 cup blueberries
- 3 ice cubes

**Preparation:**

1. Combine everything in a blender until smooth. Pour into 2 glasses and serve.

**Nutritional information:**

Calories 131, Sodium (Na) 60 mg, Protein 3 g, Potassium 146 mg, Phosphorus 51 mg, Carbs 4 g, Fat 0 g

# Peach Iced-Tea

Prep time:15 minutes, Cook time:0 minutes, Servings:2

**Ingredients:**

- 1 lemon
- 1 cup sliced canned peaches
- 1 tbsp. loose black

**Preparation:**

1. Boil a pot of water and add the peach slices.
2. Simmer for 10 minutes before turning off the heat.
3. Add the loose tea leaves and allow to steep for 5-7 minutes.
4. Pour liquid through a sieve or tea strainer.
5. Enjoy hot.

**Nutritional information:**

Calories 74, Protein 0 g, Carbs 15 g, Fat 0 g, Sodium (Na) 5 mg, Potassium (K) 15 mg, Phosphorus 14 mg

# Lemon Boost

Prep time:5 minutes, Cook time:0 minutes, Servings:2

**Ingredients:**

- 1 tsp. cinnamon
- 2 tbsps. stevia
- 1 juiced lemon
- 2 pasteurized liquid egg whites

**Preparation:**

1. Combine all ingredients in a blender until smooth.
2. Garnish with a slice of lemon and serve over ice!

**Nutritional information:**

Calories 30, Protein 3 g, Carbs 3 g, Fat 1 g, Sodium (Na)55 mg, Potassium (K) 86 mg, Phosphorus 10 mg

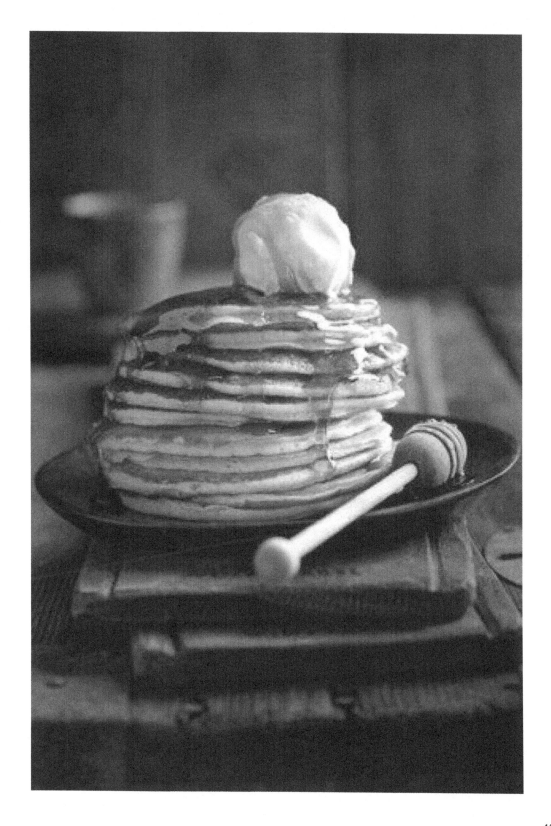

# Snacks and sides

## Mock Pancakes

Prep time:5 minutes, Cook time:5 minutes, Servings:2

**Ingredients:**

- 2 tbsps. honey
- 1 tsp. cinnamon
- 1 cup ricotta cheese
- 1 egg

**Preparation:**

1. Using a blender, put together egg, honey, cinnamon, and ricotta cheese. Process until all ingredients are well combined.
2. Pour an equal amount of the blended mixture into the pan. Cook each pancake for 4 minutes on both sides. Serve.

**Nutritional information:**

Calories 188.1, Protein 16.84g Potassium (K) 177 mg Sodium (Na) 136 mg, Fat 14.5 g, Carbs 5.5 g, Phosphorus 134 mg

# Breakfast Cheesecake

Prep time:5 minutes, Cook time:15 minutes, Servings:16

## Ingredients:

- ½ cup uncured sausage
- 2 tbsps. honey
- 7 cups cottage cheese
- Pepper, ¼ tsp.
- ½ tsp. olive oil
- 7 cups Greek yogurt
- Salt, ¼ tsp.
- 4 eggs
- 2 tsps. vanilla
- ½ chopped onion

## Preparation:

1. In a blender, combine eggs, cream cheese, cottage cheese, honey, and vanilla. Process until all ingredients are well combined.
2. Meanwhile, heat the olive oil in a pan. Saute onion and uncured sausage. Season with salt and pepper. Cook for 4 minutes. Transfer the mixture into a baking dish.
3. Place inside the oven and bake for 10 minutes. Allow to cool at room temperature. Refrigerate for 1 hour before serving.

## Nutritional information:

Protein 22.92g, Potassium (K) 244 mg, Sodium (Na) 477 mg, Phosphorus 106mg, Carbs 8.1g, Fat 6.1g, Calories 121.3

# Mock Cream Cheese Pancake

Prep time:5 minutes, Cook time:5 minutes, Servings:4

**Ingredients:**

- 1 pack Stevia
- ½ tsp. cinnamon
- 2 eggs
- 2 cups Greek yogurt

**Preparation:**

1. Put eggs, cream cheese, Stevia, and cinnamon in a blender. Process until all ingredients are well-combined.
2. Pour an equal amount of the blended mixture in a greased pan. Cook for 4 minutes on both sides. Repeat with the rest of the batter. Serve.

**Nutritional information:**

Protein 13.16g Potassium (K) 199 mg Sodium (Na) 82mg Carbs 2.5 g, Calories 289.6, Fat 26.6 g Phosphorus 282.7 mg

# Eggs Creamy Melt

Prep time:6 minutes, Cook time:4 minutes, Servings:2

**Ingredients:**

- 1 tbsp. olive oil
- Italian seasoning
- 1 cup shredded tofu
- 2 beaten eggs

**Preparation:**

1. In a small bowl, combine beaten eggs and Italian seasoning. Sprinkle tofu on top.
2. Heat the olive oil in a pan. Add the egg mixture. Cook for 4 minutes on both sides. Serve.

**Nutritional information:**

Protein 15.57g, Potassium (K) 216 mg, Sodium (Na) 107 mg, Calories 214, Fat 16.9 g, Carbs 1.4 g Phosphorous 73 mg

# Mashed Cauliflowers

Prep time:5 minutes, Cook time:5 minutes, Servings:1

**Ingredients:**

- ¼ cup sour cream
- 2 tbsps. unsalted butter
- ¼ tsp. pepper
- 1 cup cauliflower florets

**Preparation:**

1. Steam cauliflower florets for 5 minutes or until soft.
2. Process steamed florets in a food processor.
3. Add in butter and sour cream. Process again until all ingredients are well combined. Serve.

**Nutritional information:**

Protein 4.24g, Potassium (K) 448 mg, Sodium (Na) 204 mg, Calories 142, Fat 10.45g, Carbs, 8.94g, Phosphorus 68.6mg

# Banana Cookies

Prep time:4 minutes, Cook time:26 minutes, Servings:8

**Ingredients:**

- 2 tbsps. dried and chopped raisins
- 4 pitted dates
- 3 tbsps. dried and chopped cranberries
- ¼ cup unsweetened almond milk
- 1 tsp. vanilla
- 1 tsp. baking powder
- 1 tbsp. cinnamon
- 2/3 cup coconut flour
- 2 peeled ripe bananas
- 2/3 cup unsweetened applesauce
- 1 ½ tsps. lemon juice

**Preparation:**

1. Preheat the oven to 350°F.
2. In a food processor, combine almond milk, applesauce, dates, and bananas. Blend until you achieve a smooth consistency.
3. Add in coconut flour, baking powder, cinnamon, vanilla, and lemon juice. Blend for 1 minute. Fold in cranberries and raisins.
4. Pour a baking sheet with the cookie dough. Place inside the oven for 20 minutes.
5. Allow to sit for 5 minutes and let it harden. Serve.

**Nutritional information:**

Protein 1.05g, Potassium (K) 309 mg, Sodium (Na) 28 mg, Calories 64.7, Carbs 12.2 g, Fat 1.8 g, Phosphorus49.5mg

# Baked Cinnamon over Apple Raisins

Prep time:5 minutes, Cook time:5 minutes, Servings:4

**Ingredients:**

- 1 tsp. grated lemon peel
- ¼ cup raisins
- ½ tsp. ground cinnamon
- ½ cup 100% apple juice
- 2 tbsps. brown sugar
- 1/8 tsp. nutmeg
- 4 cored apples
- 1 tbsp. lemon juice

**Preparation:**

1. Layer apples in a baking dish. Fill them with raisins.
2. Meanwhile, in a small bowl, put together apple juice, nutmeg, lemon juice, ground cinnamon, brown sugar, and lemon peel. Mix ingredients until well-combined.
3. Coat apples with the mixture. Cover with plastic wrap. Set aside.
4. For the remaining cinnamon, place inside the microwave and heat for 4 minutes or until the sauce thickens.
5. Drizzle over apples Serve.

**Nutritional information:**

Protein 0.82g, Potassium (K) 303 mg, Sodium (Na) 5 mg, Calories 210, Carbs 40g, Fat 2.5g, Phosphorus 108.8mg

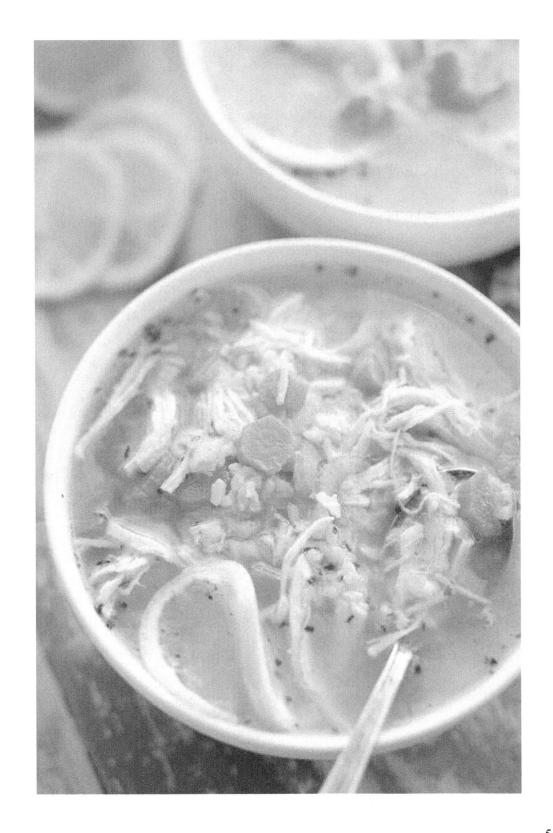

# Soups

## Spaghetti Squash & Yellow Bell-Pepper Soup

Prep time:10 minutes, Cook time:45 minutes, Servings:4

**Ingredients:**

- 2 diced yellow bell peppers
- 2 chopped large garlic cloves
- 1 peeled and cubed spaghetti squash
- 1 quartered and sliced onion
- 1 tbsp. dried thyme
- 1 tbsp. coconut oil
- 1 tsp. curry powder
- 4 cups water

**Preparation:**

1. Heat the oil in a large pan over medium-high heat before sweating the onions and garlic for 3-4 minutes.
2. Sprinkle over the curry powder.
3. Add the stock and bring to a boil over a high heat before adding the squash, pepper and thyme.
4. Turn down the heat, cover and allow to simmer for 25-30 minutes.
5. Continue to simmer until squash is soft if needed.
6. Allow to cool before blitzing in a blender/food processor until smooth.
7. Serve!

**Nutritional information:**

Calories 103, Protein 2 g, Carbs 17 g, Fat 4 g, Sodium (Na) 32 mg, Potassium (K)365 mg, Phosphorus 50 mg

# Red Pepper & Brie Soup

Prep time:10 minutes, Cook time:35 minutes, Servings:4

**Ingredients:**

- 1 tsp. paprika
- 1 tsp. cumin
- 1 chopped red onion
- 2 chopped garlic cloves
- ¼ cup crumbled brie
- 2 tbsps. extra virgin olive oil
- 4 chopped red bell peppers
- 4 cups water

**Preparation:**

1. Heat the oil in a pot over medium heat.
2. Sweat the onions and peppers for 5 minutes.
3. Add the garlic cloves, cumin and paprika and sauté for 3-4 minutes.
4. Add the water and allow to boil before turning the heat down to simmer for 30 minutes.
5. Remove from the heat and allow to cool slightly.
6. Put the mixture in a food processor and blend until smooth.
7. Pour into serving bowls and add the crumbled brie to the top with a little black pepper.
8. Enjoy!

**Nutritional information:**

Calories 152, Protein 3 g, Carbs 8 g, Fat 11 g, Sodium (Na) 66 mg, Potassium (K) 270 mg, Phosphorus 207 mg

# Turkey & Lemon-Grass Soup

Prep time:5 minutes, Cook time:40 minutes

Servings:4

**Ingredients:**

- 1 fresh lime
- ¼ cup fresh basil leaves
- 1 tbsp. cilantro
- 1 cup canned and drained water chestnuts
- 1 tbsp. coconut oil
- 1 thumb-size minced ginger piece
- 2 chopped scallions
- 1 finely chopped green chili
- 4oz. skinless and sliced turkey breasts
- 1 minced garlic clove, minced
- ½ finely sliced stick lemon-grass
- 1 chopped white onion, chopped
- 4 cups water

**Preparation:**

1. Crush the lemon-grass, cilantro, chili, 1 tbsp oil and basil leaves in a blender or pestle and mortar to form a paste.
2. Heat a large pan/wok with 1 tbsp olive oil on high heat.
3. Sauté the onions, garlic and ginger until soft.
4. Add the turkey and brown each side for 4-5 minutes.
5. Add the broth and stir.
6. Now add the paste and stir.
7. Next add the water chestnuts, turn down the heat slightly and allow to simmer for 25-30 minutes or until turkey is thoroughly cooked through.
8. Serve hot with the green onion sprinkled over the top.

**Nutritional information:**

Calories 123, Protein 10 g, Carbs 12 g, Fat 3 g, Sodium (Na) 501 mg, Potassium (K) 151 mg, Phosphorus 110 mg

# Paprika Pork Soup

Prep time:5 minutes, Cook time:35 minutes, Servings:2

## Ingredients:

- 4 oz. sliced pork loin
- 1 tsp. black pepper
- 2 minced garlic cloves
- 1 cup baby spinach
- 3 cups water
- 1 tbsp. extra-virgin olive oil
- 1 chopped onion
- 1 tbsp. paprika

## Preparation:

1. In a large pot, add the oil, chopped onion and minced garlic.
2. Sauté for 5 minutes on low heat.
3. Add the pork slices to the onions and cook for 7-8 minutes or until browned.
4. Add the water to the pan and bring to a boil on high heat.
5. Stir in the spinach, reduce heat and simmer for a further 20 minutes or until pork is thoroughly cooked through.
6. Season with pepper to serve.

## Nutritional information:

Calories 165, Protein 13 g, Carbs 10 g, Fat 9 g, Sodium (Na) 269 mg, Potassium (K) 486 mg, Phosphorus 158 mg

# Mediterranean Vegetable Soup

Prep time:5 minutes, Cook time:30 minutes, Servings:4

**Ingredients:**

- 1 tbsp. oregano
- 2 minced garlic cloves
- 1 tsp. black pepper
- 1 diced zucchini
- 1 cup diced eggplant
- 4 cups water
- 1 diced red pepper
- 1 tbsp. extra-virgin olive oil
- 1 diced red onion

**Preparation:**

1. Soak the vegetables in warm water prior to use.
2. In a large pot, add the oil, chopped onion and minced garlic.
3. Sweat for 5 minutes on low heat.
4. Add the other vegetables to the onions and cook for 7-8 minutes.
5. Add the stock to the pan and bring to a boil on high heat.
6. Stir in the herbs, reduce the heat, and simmer for a further 20 minutes or until thoroughly cooked through.
7. Season with pepper to serve.

**Nutritional information:**

Calories 152, Protein 1 g, Carbs 6 g, Fat 3 g, Sodium (Na) 3 mg, Potassium (K) 229 mg, Phosphorus 45 mg

# Tofu Soup

Prep time:5 minutes, *Cook time:* 10 minutes , Servings:2

**Ingredients:**

- 1 tbsp. miso paste
- 1/8 cup cubed soft tofu
- 1 chopped green onion
- ¼ cup sliced Shiitake mushrooms
- 3 cups Renali stock
- 1 tbsp. soy sauce

**Preparation:**

1. Take a saucepan, pour the stock into this pan and let it boil on high heat. Reduce heat to medium and let this stock simmer. Add mushrooms in this stock and cook for almost 3 minutes.
2. Take a bowl and mix Soy sauce (reduced salt) and miso paste together in this bowl. Add this mixture and tofu in stock. Simmer for nearly 5 minutes and serve with chopped green onion.

**Nutritional information:**

Calories 129, Fat 7.8g, Sodium (Na) 484mg, Potassium (K) 435mg, Protein 11g, Carbs 5.5g, Phosphorus 73.2mg

# Onion Soup

Prep time:15 minutes , Cook time:45 minutes, Servings:6

**Ingredients:**

- 2 tbsps. chicken stock
- 1 cup chopped Shiitake mushrooms
- 1 tbsp. minced chives
- 3 tsps. beef bouillon
- 1 tsp. grated ginger root
- ½ chopped carrot
- 1 cup sliced Portobello mushrooms
- 1 chopped onion
- ½ chopped celery stalk
- 2 quarts water
- ¼ tsp. minced garlic

**Preparation:**

1. Take a saucepan and combine carrot, onion, celery, garlic, mushrooms (some mushrooms) and ginger in this pan. Add water, beef bouillon and chicken stock in this pan. Put this pot on high heat and let it boil. Decrease flame to medium and cover this pan to cook for almost 45 minutes.
2. Put all remaining mushrooms in one separate pot. Once the boiling mixture is completely done, put one strainer over this new bowl with mushrooms and strain cooked soup in this pot over mushrooms. Discard solid-strained materials.
3. Serve delicious broth with yummy mushrooms in small bowls and sprinkle chives over each bowl.

**Nutritional information:**

Calories 22, Fat 0g, Sodium (Na) 602.3mg, Potassium (K) 54.1mg, Carbs 4.9g, Protein 0.6g, Phosphorus 15.8mg

# Steakhouse Soup

Prep time: 15 minutes, Cook time:25 minutes , Servings:4

**Ingredients:**

- 2 tbsps. soy sauce
- 2 boneless and cubed chicken breasts.
- ¼ lb. halved and trimmed snow peas
- 1 tbsp. minced ginger root
- 1 minced garlic clove
- 1 cup water
- 2 chopped green onions
- 3 cups chicken stock
- 1 chopped carrot
- 3 sliced mushrooms

**Preparation:**

1. Take a pot and combine ginger, water, chicken stock, Soy sauce (reduced salt) and garlic in this pot. Let them boil on medium heat, mix in chicken pieces, and let them simmer on low heat for almost 15 minutes to tender chicken.
2. Stir in carrot and snow peas and simmer for almost 5 minutes. Add mushrooms in this blend and continue cooking to tender vegetables for nearly 3 minutes. Mix in the chopped onion and serve hot.

**Nutritional information:**

Calories 319, Carbs 14g, Fat 15g, Potassium (K) 225 mg, Protein 29g, Sodium (Na) 389 mg, Phosphorous 190 mg

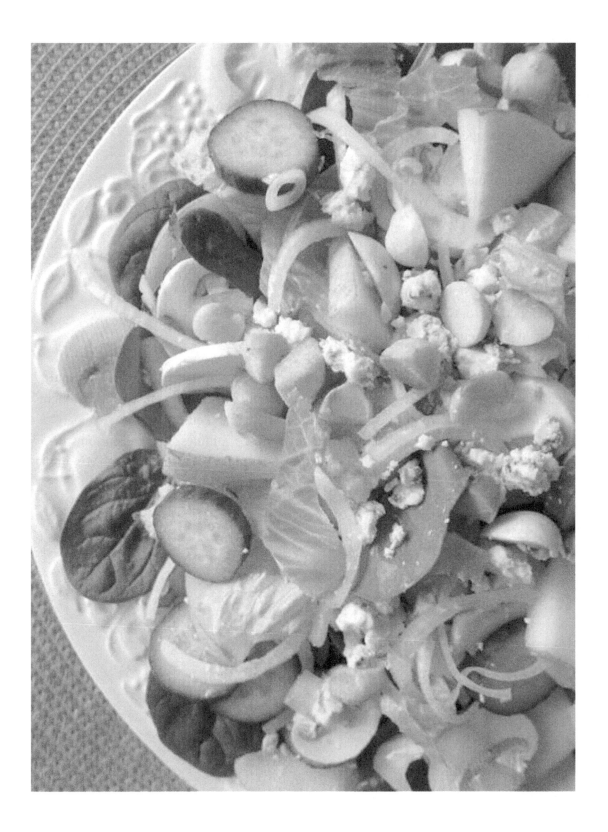

64

# Salads

## Pear & Brie Salad

Prep time:5 minutes, Cook time:0 minutes, Servings:4

**Ingredients:**

- 1 tbsp. olive oil
- 1 cup arugula
- ½ lemon
- ½ cup canned pears
- ¼ cucumber
- ¼ cup chopped brie

**Preparation:**

1. Peel and dice the cucumber.
2. Dice the pear.
3. Wash the arugula.
4. Combine salad in a serving bowl and crumble the brie over the top.
5. Whisk the olive oil and lemon juice together.
6. Drizzle over the salad.
7. Season with a little black pepper to taste and serve immediately.

**Nutritional information:**

Calories 54, Protein 1 g, Carbs 12 g, Fat 7 g, Sodium (Na) 57mg, Potassium (K) 115 mg, Phosphorus 67 mg

# Caesar Salad

Prep time:5 minutes, Cook time:5 minutes, Servings:4

**Ingredients:**

- 1 head romaine lettuce
- ¼ cup mayonnaise
- 1 tbsp. lemon juice
- 4 anchovy fillets
- 1 tsp. Worcestershire sauce
- Black pepper
- 5 garlic cloves
- 4 tbsps. Parmesan cheese
- 1 tsp. mustard

**Preparation:**

1. In a bowl mix all ingredients and mix well
2. Serve with dressing

**Nutritional information:**

Calories 44, Fat 2.1 g, Sodium (Na) 83 mg, Potassium (K) 216 mg, Carbs 4.3 g, Protein 3.2 g, Phosphorus 45.6mg

# Cucumber Salad

Prep time:5 minutes , Cook time:5 minutes , Servings:4

**Ingredients:**

- 1 tbsp. dried dill
- 1 onion
- ¼ cup water
- 1 cup vinegar
- 3 cucumbers
- ¾ cup white sugar

**Preparation:**

1. In a bowl add all ingredients and mix well
2. Serve with dressing

**Nutritional information:**

Calories 49, Fat 0.1g, Sodium (Na) 341mg, Potassium (K) 171mg, Protein 0.8g, Carbs 11g, Phosphorus 24 mg

# Thai Cucumber Salad

Prep time:5 minutes , Cook time:5 minutes , Servings:2

**Ingredients:**

- ¼ cup chopped peanuts
- ¼ cup white sugar
- ½ cup cilantro
- ¼ cup rice wine vinegar
- 3 cucumbers
- 2 jalapeno peppers

**Preparation:**

1. In a bowl add all ingredients and mix well
2. Serve with dressing

**Nutritional information:**

Calories 20, Fat 0g, Sodium (Na) 85mg, Carbs 5g, Protein 1g, Potassium (K) 190.4 mg, Phosphorus 46.8mg

# Red Potato Salad

Prep time:5 minutes , Cook time:5 minutes , Servings:2

**Ingredients:**

- 2 cups mayonnaise
- 1 lb. bacon
- 1 stalk celery
- 4 eggs
- Pepper.
- 2 lbs. red potatoes
- 1 onion

**Preparation:**

1. In a pot add water, potatoes and cook until tender
2. Remove, drain and set aside
3. Place eggs in a saucepan, add water and bring to a boil
4. Cover and let eggs stand for 10-15 minutes
5. When ready remove, meanwhile in a deep skillet cook bacon on low heat
6. In a bowl add all ingredients and mix well
7. Serve with dressing

**Nutritional information:**

Calories 280, Fat 20.0 g, Sodium (Na) 180.0 mg, Potassium (K) 0.0 mg, Carbs 26.0 g, Protein 2.0 g, Phosphorus 130mg

# Broccoli-Cauliflower Salad

Prep time:5 minutes , Cook time:5 minutes , Servings:4

**Ingredients:**

- 1 tbsp. wine vinegar
- 1 cup cauliflower florets
- ¼ cup white sugar
- 2 cups hard-cooked eggs
- 5 slices bacon
- 1 cup broccoli florets
- 1 cup cheddar cheese
- 1 cup mayonnaise

**Preparation:**

1. In a bowl add all ingredients and mix well
2. Serve with dressing

**Nutritional information:**

Calories 89.8, Fat 4.5 g, Sodium (Na) 51.2 mg, Potassium (K) 257.6 mg, Carbs 11.5 g, Protein 3.0 g, Phosphorus 47 mg

# Macaroni Salad

Prep time:5 minutes , Cook time:5 minutes , Servings:4

**Ingredients:**

- ¼ tsp. celery seed
- 2 hard-boiled eggs
- 2 cups salad dressing
- 1 onion
- 2 tsps. white vinegar
- 2 stalks celery
- 2 cups cooked macaroni
- 1 red bell pepper
- 2 tbsps. mustard

**Preparation:**

1. In a bowl add all ingredients and mix well
2. Serve with dressing

**Nutritional information:**

Calories 360, Fat 21g, Sodium (Na) 400mg, Carbs 36g, Protein 6g, Potassium (K) 68mg, Phosphorus 36 mg

# Green Bean and Potato Salad

Prep time:5 minutes, Cook time:5 minutes, Servings:4

**Ingredients:**

- ½ cup basil
- ¼ cup olive oil
- 1 tbsp. mustard
- ¾ lb. green beans
- 1 tbsp. lemon juice
- ½ cup balsamic vinegar
- 1 red onion
- 1 lb. red potatoes
- 1 garlic clove

**Preparation:**

1. Place potatoes in a pot with water and bring to a boil for 15-18 minutes or until tender
2. Thrown in green beans after 5-6 minutes
3. Drain and cut into cubes
4. In a bowl add all ingredients and mix well
5. Serve with dressing

**Nutritional information:**

Calories 153.2, Fat 2.0 g, Sodium (Na) 77.6 mg, Potassium (K) 759.0 mg, Carbs 29.0 g, Protein 6.9 g, Phosphorus 49 mg

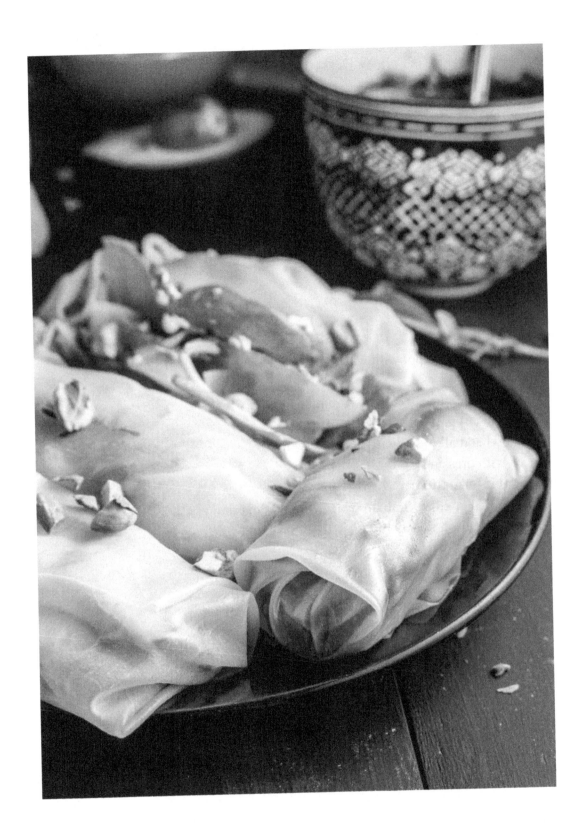

# Vegetables

## Thai Tofu Broth

Prep time:5 minutes, Cook time:15 minutes, Servings:4

**Ingredients:**

- 1 cup rice noodles
- ½ sliced onion
- 6 oz. drained, pressed and cubed tofu
- ¼ cup sliced scallions
- ½ cup water
- ½ cup canned water chestnuts
- ½ cup rice milk
- 1 tbsp. lime juice
- 1 tbsp. coconut oil
- ½ finely sliced chili
- 1 cup snow peas

**Preparation:**

1. Heat the oil in a wok on a high heat and then sauté the tofu until brown on each side.
2. Add the onion and sauté for 2-3 minutes.
3. Add the rice milk and water to the wok until bubbling.
4. Lower to medium heat and add the noodles, chili and water chestnuts.
5. Allow to simmer for 10-15 minutes and then add the sugar snap peas for 5 minutes.
6. Serve with a sprinkle of scallions.

**Nutritional information:**

Calories 304, Protein 9 g, Carbs 38 g, Fat 13 g, Sodium (Na) 36 mg, Potassium (K) 114 mg, Phosphorus 101 mg

# Delicious Vegetarian Lasagne

Prep time:10 minutes, Cook time:1 hour , Servings:4

**Ingredients:**

- 1 tsp. basil
- 1 tbsp. olive oil
- ½ sliced red pepper
- 3 lasagna sheets
- ½ diced red onion
- ¼ tsp. black pepper
- 1 cup rice milk
- 1 minced garlic clove
- 1 cup sliced eggplant
- ½ sliced zucchini
- ½ pack soft tofu
- 1 tsp. oregano

**Preparation:**

1. Preheat oven to 325°F/Gas Mark 3.
2. Slice zucchini, eggplant and pepper into vertical strips.
3. Add the rice milk and tofu to a food processor and blitz until smooth. Set aside.
4. Heat the oil in a skillet over medium heat and add the onions and garlic for 3-4 minutes or until soft.
5. Sprinkle in the herbs and pepper and allow to stir through for 5-6 minutes until hot.
6. Into a lasagne or suitable oven dish, layer 1 lasagna sheet, then 1/3 the eggplant, followed by 1/3 zucchini, then 1/3 pepper before pouring over 1/3 of tofu white sauce.
7. Repeat for the next 2 layers, finishing with the white sauce.
8. Add to the oven for 40-50 minutes or until veg is soft and can easily be sliced into servings.

**Nutritional information:**

Calories 235, Protein 5 g, Carbs 10g, Fat 9 g, Sodium (Na) 35 mg, Potassium (K) 129 mg, Phosphorus 66 mg

# Chili Tofu Noodles

Prep time:5 minutes, Cook time:15 minutes, Servings:4

## Ingredients:

- ½ diced red chili
- 2 cups rice noodles
- ½ juiced lime
- 6 oz. pressed and cubed silken firm tofu
- 1 tsp. grated fresh ginger
- 1 tbsp. coconut oil
- 1 cup green beans
- 1 minced garlic clove

## Preparation:

1. Steam the green beans for 10-12 minutes or according to package directions and drain.
2. Cook the noodles in a pot of boiling water for 10-15 minutes or according to package directions.
3. Meanwhile, heat a wok or skillet on a high heat and add coconut oil.
4. Now add the tofu, chili flakes, garlic and ginger and sauté for 5-10 minutes.
5. Drain the noodles and add to the wok along with the green beans and lime juice.
6. Toss to coat.
7. Serve hot!

## Nutritional information:

Calories 246, Protein 10 g, Carbs 28g, Fat 12 g, Sodium (Na) 25 mg, Potassium (K) 126 mg, Phosphorus 79 mg

# Curried Cauliflower

Prep time:5 minutes, Cook time:20 minutes, Servings:4

## Ingredients:

- 1 tsp. turmeric
- 1 diced onion
- 1 tbsp chopped fresh cilantro
- 1 tsp. cumin
- ½ diced chili
- ½ cup water
- 1 minced garlic clove
- 1 tbsp. coconut oil
- 1 tsp. garam masala
- 2 cups cauliflower florets

## Preparation:

1. Add the oil to a skillet on medium heat.
2. Sauté the onion and garlic for 5 minutes until soft.
3. Add the cumin, turmeric and garam masala and stir to release the aromas.
4. Now add the chili to the pan along with the cauliflower.
5. Stir to coat.
6. Pour in the water and reduce the heat to a simmer for 15 minutes.
7. Garnish with cilantro to serve.

## Nutritional information:

Calories 108, Protein 2 g, Carbs 11 g, Fat 7 g, Sodium (Na) 35 mg, Potassium (K) 328 mg, Phosphorus 39 mg

# Chinese Tempeh Stir Fry

Prep time:5 minutes, Cook time:15 minutes, Servings:2

**Ingredients:**

- 2 oz. sliced tempeh
- 1 cup cooked brown rice
- 1 minced garlic clove
- ½ cup green onions
- 1 tsp. minced fresh ginger
- 1 tbsp. coconut oil
- ½ cup corn

**Preparation:**

1. Heat the oil in a skillet or wok on a high heat and add the garlic and ginger.
2. Sauté for 1 minute.
3. Now add the tempeh and cook for 5-6 minutes before adding the corn for a further 10 minutes.
4. Now add the green onions and serve over brown rice.

**Nutritional information:**

Calories 304, Protein 10 g, Carbs 35 g, Fat 4 g, Sodium (Na) 91 mg, Potassium (K) 121 mg, Phosphorus 222 mg

# Parsley Root Veg Stew

Prep time:5 minutes, Cook time:35-40 minutes, Servings:4

**Ingredients:**

- 2 garlic cloves
- 2 cups white rice
- 1 tsp. ground cumin
- 1 diced onion
- 2 cups water
- 4 peeled and diced turnips
- 1 tsp. cayenne pepper
- ¼ cup chopped fresh parsley
- ½ tsp. ground cinnamon
- 2 tbsps. olive oil
- 1 tsp. ground ginger
- 2 peeled and diced carrots

**Preparation:**

1. In a large pot, heat the oil on a medium high heat before sautéing the onion for 4-5 minutes until soft.
2. Add the turnips and cook for 10 minutes or until golden brown.
3. Add the garlic, cumin, ginger, cinnamon, and cayenne pepper, cooking for a further 3 minutes.
4. Add the carrots and stock to the pot and then bring to the boil.
5. Turn the heat down to medium heat, cover and simmer for 20 minutes.
6. Meanwhile add the rice to a pot of water and bring to the boil.
7. Turn down to simmer for 15 minutes.
8. Drain and place the lid on for 5 minutes to steam.
9. Garnish the root vegetable stew with parsley to serve alongside the rice.

**Nutritional information:**

Calories 210, Protein 4 g, Carbs 32 g, Fat 7 g, Sodium (Na) 67 mg, Potassium (K) 181 mg, Phosphorus 105 mg

# Mixed Pepper Paella

Prep time:10 minutes, Cook time:35-40 minutes, Servings:2

**Ingredients:**

- 1 tbsp. extra virgin olive oil
- ½ chopped red onion
- 1 lemon
- ½ chopped yellow bell pepper
- 1 cup homemade chicken broth
- ½ chopped zucchini
- 1 tsp. dried oregano
- ½ chopped red bell pepper
- 1 tsp. dried parsley
- 1 cup brown rice
- 1 tsp. paprika

**Preparation:**

1. Add the rice to a pot of cold water and cook for 15 minutes.
2. Drain the water, cover the pan and leave to one side.
3. Heat the oil in a skillet over medium-high heat.
4. Add the bell peppers, onion and zucchini, sautéing for 5 minutes.
5. To the pan, add the rice, herbs, spices and juice of the lemon along with the chicken broth.
6. Cover and turn the heat right down and allow to simmer for 15-20 minutes.
7. Serve hot.

**Nutritional information:**

Calories 210, Protein 4 g, Carbs 33 g, Fat 7 g, Sodium (Na) 20 mg, Potassium (K) 33 mg, Phosphorus 156 mg

# Cauliflower Rice & Runny Eggs

Prep time:5 minutes, Cook time:30 minutes, Servings:4

## Ingredients:

- 4 eggs
- 1 tbsp. extra virgin olive oil
- 1 tsp. black pepper
- 1 tbsp. chopped fresh chives
- 2 cups cauliflower
- 1 tbsp. curry powder

## Preparation:

1. Preheat the oven to 375°F/Gas Mark 5.
2. Soak the cauliflower in warm water in advance if possible.
3. Grate or chop into rice-size pieces.
4. Bring the cauliflower to the boil in a pot of water and then turn down to simmer for 7 minutes.
5. Drain completely.
6. Place on a baking tray and sprinkle over curry powder and black pepper - toss to coat.
7. Bake in the oven for 20 minutes, stirring occasionally.
8. Meanwhile, boil a separate pan of water and add the eggs for 7 minutes.
9. Run under the cold tap, crack and peel the eggs before cutting in half.
10. Top the cauliflower with eggs and chopped chives.
11. Serve hot!

## Nutritional information:

Calories 120, Protein 7 g, Carbs 4 g, Fat 8 g, Sodium (Na) 175 mg, Potassium (K) 188 mg, Phosphorus 134 mg

# Minted Zucchini Noodles

Prep time:5 minutes, Cook time:10 minutes, Servings:2

**Ingredients:**

- ¼ deseeded and chopped red chili
- 2 tbsps. Extra virgin olive oil
- ½ juiced lemon
- 4 peeled and sliced zucchinis
- ½ cup chopped fresh mint
- 1 tsp. black pepper
- ½ cup arugula

**Preparation:**

1. Whisk the mint, pepper, chili and olive oil to make a dressing.
2. Meanwhile, heat a pan of water on a high heat and bring to the boil.
3. Add the zucchini noodles and turn the heat down to simmer for 3-4 minutes.
4. Remove from the heat and place in a bowl of cold water immediately.
5. Toss the noodles in the dressing.
6. Mix the arugula with the lemon juice to serve on the top.
7. Enjoy!

**Nutritional information:**

Calories 148, Protein 2 g, Carbs 4 g, Fat 13 g, Sodium (Na) 7 mg, Potassium (K) 422 mg, Phosphorus 256 mg

# Chili Tempeh & Scallions

Prep time:10 minutes, Cook time:15 minutes, Servings:2

**Ingredients:**

- ½ cup chopped scallions
- 1 juiced lime
- 1 tsp. soy sauce
- 2 oz. cubed tempeh
- 1 tbsp. grated ginger
- 1 tsp. coconut oil
- ½ deseeded and chopped red chili

**Preparation:**

1. Mix the oil, soy sauce, chili flakes, lime juice and ginger together.
2. Marinate the tempeh in this for as long as possible.
3. Preheat the broiler to medium heat.
4. Add tempeh to a lined baking tray and broil for 10-15 minutes or until hot through.
5. Remove and sprinkle with scallions to serve.

**Nutritional information:**

Calories 221, Protein 6 g, Carbs 8 g, Fat 10 g, Sodium (Na) 466 mg, Potassium (K) 189 mg, Phosphorus 99 mg

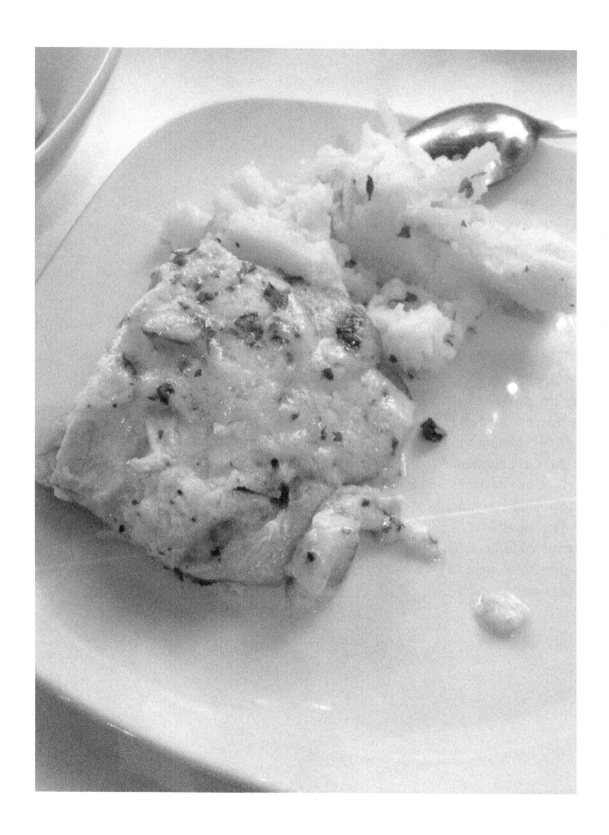

# Seafood

## Shrimp Paella

Prep time:5 minutes, Cook time:10 minutes, Servings:2

**Ingredients:**

- 1 cup cooked brown rice
- 1 chopped red onion
- 1 tsp. paprika
- 1 chopped garlic clove
- 1 tbsp. olive oil
- 6 oz. frozen cooked shrimp
- 1 deseeded and sliced chili pepper
- 1 tbsp. oregano

**Preparation:**

1. Heat the olive oil in a large pan on medium-high heat.
2. Add the onion and garlic and sauté for 2-3 minutes until soft.
3. Now add the shrimp and sauté for a further 5 minutes or until hot through.
4. Now add the herbs, spices, chili and rice with 1/2 cup boiling water.
5. Stir until everything is warm and the water has been absorbed.
6. Plate up and serve.

**Nutritional information:**

Calories 221 Protein 17 g Carbs 31 g Fat 8 g Sodium (Na) 235 mg Potassium (K) 176 mg Phosphorus 189 mg

# Salmon & Pesto Salad

Prep time:5 minutes, Cook time:15 minutes, Servings:2

**Ingredients:**

**For the pesto:**

- 1 minced garlic clove
- ½ cup fresh arugula
- ¼ cup extra virgin olive oil
- ½ cup fresh basil
- 1 tsp. black pepper

**For the salmon:**

- 4 oz. skinless salmon fillet
- 1 tbsp. coconut oil

**For the salad:**

- ½ juiced lemon
- 2 sliced radishes
- ½ cup iceberg lettuce
- 1 tsp. black pepper

**Preparation:**

1. Prepare the pesto by blending all the ingredients for the pesto in a food processor or by grinding with a pestle and mortar. Set aside.
2. Add a skillet to the stove on medium-high heat and melt the coconut oil.
3. Add the salmon to the pan.
4. Cook for 7-8 minutes and turn over.
5. Cook for a further 3-4 minutes or until cooked through.
6. Remove fillets from the skillet and allow to rest.
7. Mix the lettuce and the radishes and squeeze over the juice of ½ lemon.
8. Flake the salmon with a fork and mix through the salad.
9. Toss to coat and sprinkle with a little black pepper to serve.

**Nutritional information:**

Calories 221, Protein 13 g, Carbs 1 g, Fat 34 g, Sodium (Na) 80 mg, Potassium (K) 119 mg, Phosphorus 158 mg

# Baked Fennel & Garlic Sea Bass

Prep time:5 minutes, Cook time:15 minutes, Servings:2

**Ingredients:**

- 1 lemon
- ½ sliced fennel bulb
- 6 oz. sea bass fillets
- 1 tsp. black pepper
- 2 garlic cloves

**Preparation:**

1. Preheat the oven to 375°F/Gas Mark 5.
2. Sprinkle black pepper over the Sea Bass.
3. Slice the fennel bulb and garlic cloves.
4. Add 1 salmon fillet and half the fennel and garlic to one sheet of baking paper or tin foil.
5. Squeeze in 1/2 lemon juices.
6. Repeat for the other fillet.
7. Fold and add to the oven for 12-15 minutes or until fish is thoroughly cooked through.
8. Meanwhile, add boiling water to your couscous, cover and allow to steam.
9. Serve with your choice of rice or salad.

**Nutritional information:**

Calories 221, Protein 14 g, Carbs 3 g, Fat 2 g, Sodium (Na) 119 mg, Potassium (K) 398 mg, Phosphorus 149 mg

# Lemon, Garlic & Cilantro Tuna and Rice

Prep time:5 minutes, Cook time:0 minutes, Servings:2

## Ingredients:

- ½ cup arugula
- 1 tbsp. extra virgin olive oil
- 1 cup cooked rice
- 1 tsp. black pepper
- ¼ finely diced red onion
- 1 juiced lemon
- 3 oz. canned tuna
- 2 tbsps. Chopped fresh cilantro

## Preparation:

1. Mix the olive oil, pepper, cilantro and red onion in a bowl.
2. Stir in the tuna, cover and leave in the fridge for as long as possible (if you can) or serve immediately.
3. When ready to eat, serve up with the cooked rice and arugula!

## Nutritional information:

Calories 221, Protein 11 g, Carbs 26 g, Fat 7 g, Sodium (Na) 143 mg, Potassium (K)197 mg, Phosphorus 182 mg

# Cod & Green Bean Risotto

Prep time:4 minutes, Cook time:40 minutes, Servings:2

**Ingredients:**

- ½ cup arugula
- 1 finely diced white onion
- 4 oz. cod fillet
- 1 cup white rice
- 2 lemon wedges
- 1 cup boiling water
- ¼ tsp. black pepper
- 1 cup low sodium chicken broth
- 1 tbsp. extra virgin olive oil
- ½ cup green beans

**Preparation:**

1. Heat the oil in a large pan on medium heat.
2. Sauté the chopped onion for 5 minutes until soft before adding in the rice and stirring for 1-2 minutes.
3. Combine the broth with boiling water.
4. Add half of the liquid to the pan and stir slowly.
5. Slowly add the rest of the liquid whilst continuously stirring for up to 20-30 minutes.
6. Stir in the green beans to the risotto.
7. Place the fish on top of the rice, cover and steam for 10 minutes.
8. Ensure the water does not dry out and keep topping up until the rice is cooked thoroughly.
9. Use your fork to break up the fish fillets and stir into the rice.
10. Sprinkle with freshly ground pepper to serve and a squeeze of fresh lemon.
11. Garnish with the lemon wedges and serve with the arugula.

**Nutritional information:**

Calories 221, Protein 12 g, Carbs 29 g, Fat 8 g, Sodium (Na) 398 mg, Potassium (K) 347 mg, Phosphorus 241 mg

# Mixed Pepper Stuffed River Trout

Prep time:5 minutes, Cook time:20 minutes, Servings:4

**Ingredients:**

- 1 whole river trout
- 1 tsp. thyme
- ¼ diced yellow pepper
- 1 cup baby spinach leaves
- ¼ diced green pepper
- 1 juiced lime
- ¼ diced red pepper
- 1 tsp. oregano
- 1 tsp. extra virgin olive oil
- 1 tsp. black pepper

**Preparation:**

1. Preheat the broiler /grill on high heat.
2. Lightly oil a baking tray.
3. Mix all of the ingredients apart from the trout and lime.
4. Slice the trout lengthways (there should be an opening here from where it was gutted) and stuff the mixed ingredients inside.
5. Squeeze the lime juice over the fish and then place the lime wedges on the tray.
6. Place under the broiler on the baking tray and broil for 15-20 minutes or until fish is thoroughly cooked through and flakes easily.
7. Enjoy alone or with a side helping of rice or salad.

**Nutritional information:**

Calories 290, Protein 15 g, Carbs 0 g, Fat 7 g, Sodium (Na) 43 mg, Potassium (K) 315 mg, Phosphorus 189 mg

# Haddock & Buttered Leeks

Prep time:5 minutes, Cook time:15 minutes, Servings:2

**Ingredients:**

- 1 tbsp. unsalted butter
- 1 sliced leek
- ¼ tsp. black pepper
- 2 tsps. Chopped parsley
- 6 oz. haddock fillets
- ½ juiced lemon

**Preparation:**

1. Preheat the oven to 375°F/Gas Mark 5.
2. Add the haddock fillets to baking or parchment paper and sprinkle with the black pepper.
3. Squeeze over the lemon juice and wrap into a parcel.
4. Bake the parcel on a baking tray for 10-15 minutes or until fish is thoroughly cooked through.
5. Meanwhile, heat the butter over medium-low heat in a small pan.
6. Add the leeks and parsley and sauté for 5-7 minutes until soft.
7. Serve the haddock fillets on a bed of buttered leeks and enjoy!

**Nutritional information:**

Calories 124, Protein 15 g, Carbs 0 g, Fat 7 g, Sodium (Na) 161 mg, Potassium (K) 251 mg, Phosphorus 220 mg

# Thai Spiced Halibut

Prep time:5 minutes, Cook time:20 minutes, Servings:2

**Ingredients:**

- 2 tbsps. coconut oil
- 1 cup white rice
- ¼ tsp. black pepper
- ½ diced red chili
- 1 tbsp. fresh basil
- 2 pressed garlic cloves
- 4 oz. halibut fillet
- 1 halved lime
- 2 sliced green onions
- 1 lime leaf

**Preparation:**

1. Preheat oven to 400°F/Gas Mark 5.
2. Add half of the ingredients into baking paper and fold into a parcel.
3. Repeat for your second parcel.
4. Add to the oven for 15-20 minutes or until fish is thoroughly cooked through.
5. Serve with cooked rice.

**Nutritional information:**

Calories 311, Protein 16 g, Carbs 17 g, Fat 15 g, Sodium (Na) 31 mg, Potassium (K) 418 mg, Phosphorus 257 mg

# Homemade Tuna Nicoise

Prep time:5 minutes, Cook time:10 minutes, Servings:2

## Ingredients:

- 1 egg
- ½ cup green beans
- ¼ sliced cucumber
- 1 juiced lemon
- 1 tsp. black pepper
- ¼ sliced red onion
- 1 tbsp. olive oil
- 1 tbsp. capers
- 4 oz. drained canned tuna
- 4 iceberg lettuce leaves
- 1 tsp. chopped fresh cilantro

## Preparation:

1. Prepare the salad by washing and slicing the lettuce, cucumber and onion.
2. Add to a salad bowl.
3. Mix 1 tbsp oil with the lemon juice, cilantro and capers for a salad dressing. Set aside.
4. Boil a pan of water on high heat then lower to simmer and add the egg for 6 minutes. (Steam the green beans over the same pan in a steamer/colander for the 6 minutes).
5. Remove the egg and rinse under cold water.
6. Peel before slicing in half.
7. Mix the tuna, salad and dressing together in a salad bowl.
8. Toss to coat.
9. Top with the egg and serve with a sprinkle of black pepper.

## Nutritional information:

Calories 199, Protein 19 g, Carbs 7 g, Fat 8 g, Sodium (Na) 466 mg, Potassium (K) 251 mg, Phosphorus 211 mg

# Monk-Fish Curry

Prep time:5 minutes, Cook time:20 minutes, Servings:2

**Ingredients:**

- 1 garlic clove
- 3 finely chopped green onions
- 1 tsp. grated ginger
- 1 cup water.
- 2 tsps. Chopped fresh basil
- 1 cup cooked rice noodles
- 1 tbsp. coconut oil
- ½ sliced red chili
- 4 oz. Monk-fish fillet
- ½ finely sliced stick lemon-grass
- 2 tbsps. chopped shallots

**Preparation:**

1. Slice the Monk-fish into bite-size pieces.
2. Using a pestle and mortar or food processor, crush the basil, garlic, ginger, chili and lemon-grass to form a paste.
3. Heat the oil in a large wok or pan over medium-high heat and add the shallots.
4. Now add the water to the pan and bring to the boil.
5. Add the Monk-fish, lower the heat and cover to simmer for 10 minutes or until cooked through.
6. Enjoy with rice noodles and scatter with green onions to serve.

**Nutritional information:**

Calories 249, Protein 12 g, Carbs 30 g, Fat 10 g, Sodium (Na) 32 mg, Potassium (K) 398 mg, Phosphorus 190 mg

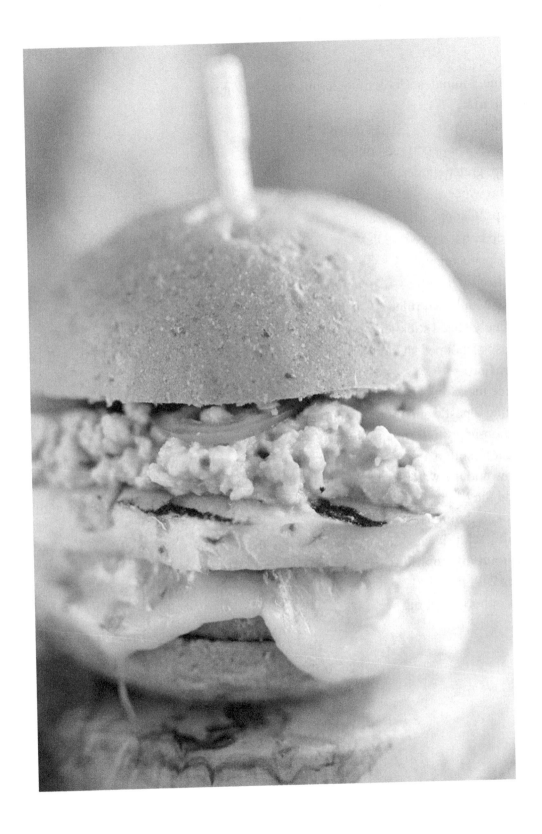

# Poultry And Meat

## Grilled Spiced Turkey

Prep time:5 minutes, Cook time:20 minutes, Servings:4

**Ingredients:**

- 6 oz. skinless and sliced turkey breast
- 1 tsp. cinnamon
- 1 tsp. curry powder
- 1 tbsp. olive oil
- 1 tsp. nutmeg

**Preparation:**

1. Whisk the oil and spices together and baste the turkey slices, coating thoroughly.
2. Cover and leave to marinade for as long as possible (ideally overnight).
3. When ready to cook, preheat the broiler to a medium-high heat and layer the turkey slices on a baking tray.
4. Place under the broiler for 15-20 minutes or according to package directions.
5. Turn occasionally.

**Nutritional information:**

Calories 101, Protein 9 g, Carbs 6 g, Fat 11 g, Sodium (Na) 42 mg, Potassium (K) 27 mg, Phosphorus 102 mg

# Her by Chicken Stew

Prep time:5 minutes, Cook time:40 minutes, Servings:6

**Ingredients:**

- 10 oz. skinless and diced chicken breast
- ½ cup white rice
- ½ diced red onion
- 1 tsp. dried oregano
- 1 tsp. dried thyme
- 1 tsp. olive oil
- ½ cup diced eggplant
- Black pepper
- 1 cup water

**Preparation:**

1. Soak vegetables in warm water prior to use if possible.
2. Heat an oven-proof pot over medium-high heat and add olive oil.
3. Add the diced chicken breast and brown in the pot for 5-6 minutes, stirring to brown each side.
4. Once the chicken is browned, lower the heat to medium and add the vegetables to the pot to sauté for 5-6 minutes - careful not to let the vegetables brown.
5. Add the water, herbs and pepper and bring to the boil.
6. Reduce the heat and simmer (lid on) for 30-40 minutes or until chicken is thoroughly cooked through.
7. Meanwhile, prepare your rice by rinsing in cold water first and then adding to a pan of cold water and bringing to the boil over high heat.
8. Reduce the heat to medium and cook for 15 minutes.
9. Drain the rice and add back to the pan with the lid on to steam until the stew is ready.
10. Serve the stew on a bed of rice and enjoy!

**Nutritional information:**

Calories 143, Protein 15 g, Carbs 9 g, Fat 5 g, Sodium (Na) 12 mg, Potassium (K) 20 mg, Phosphorus 153 mg

# Lemon & Herb Chicken Wraps

Prep time:5 minutes, Cook time:30 minutes, Servings:4

**Ingredients:**

- 4 oz. skinless and sliced chicken breasts
- ½ sliced red bell pepper
- 1 lemon
- 4 large iceberg lettuce leaves
- 1 tbsp. olive oil
- 2 tbsps. Finely chopped fresh cilantro
- ¼ tsp. black pepper

**Preparation:**

1. Preheat the oven to 375°F/Gas Mark 5.
2. Mix the oil, juice of ½ lemon, cilantro and black pepper.
3. Marinate the chicken in the oil marinade, cover and leave in the fridge for as long as possible.
4. Wrap the chicken in parchment paper, drizzling over the remaining marinade.
5. Place in the oven in an oven dish for 25-30 minutes or until chicken is thoroughly cooked through and white inside.
6. Divide the sliced bell pepper and layer onto each lettuce leaf.
7. Divide the chicken onto each lettuce leaf and squeeze over the remaining lemon juice to taste.
8. Season with a little extra black pepper if desired.
9. Wrap and enjoy!

**Nutritional information:**

Calories 200, Protein 9 g, Carbs 5 g, Fat 13 g, Sodium (Na) 25 mg, Potassium (K) 125 mg, Phosphorus 81 mg

# Ginger & Bean Sprout Steak Stir-Fry

Prep time:4 minutes, Cook time:10 minutes, Servings:2

**Ingredients:**

- 2 tsps. Grated fresh ginger
- 1 tsp. coconut oil
- 1 tsp. nutmeg
- 1 finely sliced green onion
- ¼ cup bean sprouts
- 5 oz. sliced lean organic beef steak
- 1 minced garlic clove

**Preparation:**

1. Slice the beef into strips and add to a dry hot pan, cooking for 4-5 minutes on each side or until they're cooked to your liking. Set aside.
2. Add the oil to a clean pan and sauté the bean sprouts and onions with the ginger, garlic and nutmeg for 1 minute.
3. Serve the beef strips on a bed of the vegetables and enjoy.

**Nutritional information:**

Calories 227, Protein 13 g, Carbs 13 g, Fat 23 g, Sodium (Na) 50 mg, Potassium (K) 258 mg, Phosphorus 170 mg

# Carrot & Ginger Chicken Noodles

Prep time:5 minutes, Cook time:10 minutes, Servings:4

**Ingredients:**

- 1 sliced green onion
- 2 tsps. grated fresh ginger
- 4 oz. skinless sliced chicken breasts
- 1 lime
- 1 minced garlic clove
- 1 cup cooked rice noodles
- 1 tsp. coconut oil
- 1 peeled and grated carrot

**Preparation:**

1. Heat a wok or large pan over medium-high heat.
2. Add the coconut oil to a pan and once melted, add the sliced chicken and brown for 4-5 minutes.
3. Now add the ginger and garlic and sauté for 4-5 minutes.
4. Add the green onion, carrot and lime juice to the wok.
5. Add the cooked noodles to the wok and toss until hot through.
6. Serve piping hot and enjoy.

**Nutritional information:**

Calories 187, Protein 11 g, Carbs 25 g, Fat 5 g, Sodium (Na) 39 mg, Potassium (K) 91 mg, Phosphorus 178 mg

# Roast Beef

Prep time:25 minutes , Cook time:55 minutes ,Serves:3

**Ingredients:**

• Quality rump or sirloin tip roast

**Preparation:**

1. Place in roasting pan on a shallow rack
2. Season with pepper and herbs
3. Insert meat thermometer in the center or thickest part of the roast
4. Roast to the desired degree of doneness
5. After removing from over for about 15 minutes let it chill
6. In the end the roast should be moister than well done.

**Nutritional information:**

Calories 158, Protein 24 g, Fat 6 g, Carbs 0 g, Phosphorus 206 mg, Potassium (K) 328 mg Sodium (Na) 55 mg

# Beef Brochettes

Prep time:20 minutes , Cook time:60 minutes , Servings:1

**Ingredients:**

- 1 ½ cups pineapple chunks
- 1 sliced large onion
- 2 lbs. thick steak
- 1 sliced medium bell pepper

**For the marinade:**

- 1 bay leaf
- ¼ cup vegetable oil
- ½ cup lemon juice
- 2 crushed garlic cloves

**Preparation:**

1. Cut beef cubes and place in a plastic bag
2. Combine marinade ingredients in small bowl
3. Mix and pour over beef cubes
4. Seal the bag and refrigerate for 3 to 5 hours
5. Divide ingredients:onion, beef cube, green pepper, pineapple
6. Grill about 9 minutes each side

**Nutritional information:**

Calories 304, Protein 35 g, Fat 15 g, Carbs 11 g, Phosphorus 264 mg, Potassium (K) 388 mg, Sodium (Na) 70 mg

# Country Fried Steak

Prep time:10 minutes , Cook time:100 minutes , Servings:3

**Ingredients:**

- 1 large onion
- ½ cup flour
- 3 tbsps. vegetable oil
- ¼ tsp. pepper
- 1½ lbs. round steak
- ½ tsp. paprika

**Preparation:**

1. Trim excess fat from steak
2. Cut into small pieces
3. Combine flour, paprika and pepper and mix together
4. Preheat skillet with oil
5. Cook steak on both sides
6. When the color of steak is brown remove to a platter
7. Add water (150 ml) and stir around the skillet
8. Return browned steak to skillet, if necessary, add water again so that bottom side of steak does not stick

**Nutritional information:**

Calories 248, Protein 30 g, Fat 10 g, Carbs 5 g, Phosphorus 190 mg, Potassium (K) 338 mg, Sodium (Na) 60 mg

# Beef Pot Roast

Prep time:20 minutes , Cook time:60 minutes , Servings:3

**Ingredients:**

- Round bone roast
- 2 - 4 lbs. chuck roast

**Preparation:**

1. Trim off excess fat
2. Place a tablespoon of oil in a large skillet and heat to medium
3. Roll pot roast in flour and brown on all sides in a hot skillet
4. After the meat gets a brown color, reduce heat to low
5. Season with pepper and herbs and add ½ cup of water
6. Cook slowly for 1½ hours or until it looks ready

**Nutritional information:**

Calories 157, Protein 24 g, Fat 13 g, Carbs 0 g, Phosphorus 204 mg, Potassium (K) 328 mg, Sodium (Na) 50 mg

# Meat Loaf

Prep time:20 minutes , Cook time:20 minutes , Servings:1

**Ingredients:**

- ½ tsp. ground sage
- 1 egg
- ¼ tsp. garlic powder
- 1 cup milk
- 1 tbsp. chopped parsley
- 4 soft bread slices
- ½ lb. lean ground pork
- ¼ tsp. pepper
- ¼ tsp. mustard
- 1 lb. lean ground beef
- ¼ cup onion

**Preparation:**

1. Heat oven at 350 °F
2. Mix elements in a bowl
3. Place mixture in a shallow baking dish
4. Bake ½ hours or until done (At the end loaf should be crispy brown)

**Nutritional information:**

Calories 261, Protein 27 g, Fat 12 g, Carbs 8 g, Phosphorus 244 mg, Potassium (K) 450 mg, Sodium (Na) 180 mg

# Spiced Lamb Burgers

Prep time:10 minutes, Cook time:20 minutes, Servings:2

**Ingredients:**

- 1 tbsp. extra virgin olive oil
- 1 tsp. cumin
- ½ finely diced red onion
- 1 minced garlic clove
- 1 tsp. harissa spices
- 1 cup arugula
- 1 juiced lemon
- 6 oz. lean ground lamb
- 1 tbsp. parsley
- ½ cup low-fat plain yogurt

**Preparation:**

1. Preheat the broiler on a medium to high heat.
2. Mix together the ground lamb, red onion, parsley, Harissa spices and olive oil until combined.
3. Shape 1-inch thick patties using wet hands.
4. Add the patties to a baking tray and place under the broiler for 7-8 minutes on each side or until thoroughly cooked through.
5. Mix the yogurt, lemon juice and cumin and serve over the lamb burgers with a side salad of arugula.

**Nutritional information:**

Calories 306, Fat 20g, Carbs 10g, Phosphorus 269mg, Potassium (K) 492mg, Sodium (Na) 86mg, Protein 23g

# Pork Loins with Leeks

Prep time:10 minutes, Cook time:35 minutes, Servings:2

## Ingredients:

- 1 sliced leek
- 1 tbsp. mustard seeds
- 6 oz. Pork tenderloin
- 1 tbsp. cumin seeds
- 1 tbsp. dry mustard
- 1 tbsp. extra virgin oil

## Preparation:

1. Preheat the broiler to medium high heat.
2. In a dry skillet heat mustard and cumin seeds until they start to pop (3-5 minutes).
3. Grind seeds using a pestle and mortar or blender and then mix in the dry mustard.
4. Coat the pork on both sides with the mustard blend and add to a baking tray to broil for 25-30 minutes or until cooked through. Turn once halfway through.
5. Remove and place to one side.
6. Heat the oil in a pan on medium heat and add the leeks for 5-6 minutes or until soft.
7. Serve the pork tenderloin on a bed of leeks and enjoy!

## Nutritional information:

Calories 139, Fat 5g, Carbs 2g, Phosphorus 278mg, Potassium (K) 45mg, Sodium (Na) 47mg, Protein 18g

# Chinese Beef Wraps

Prep time:10 minutes, Cook time:30 minutes, Servings:2

**Ingredients:**

- 2 iceberg lettuce leaves
- ½ diced cucumber
- 1 tsp. canola oil
- 5 oz. lean ground beef
- 1 tsp. ground ginger
- 1 tbsp. chili flakes
- 1 minced garlic clove
- 1 tbsp. rice wine vinegar

**Preparation:**

1. Mix the ground meat with the garlic, rice wine vinegar, chili flakes and ginger in a bowl.
2. Heat oil in a skillet over medium heat.
3. Add the beef to the pan and cook for 20-25 minutes or until cooked through.
4. Serve beef mixture with diced cucumber in each lettuce wrap and fold.

**Nutritional information:**

Calories 156, Fat 2g, Carbs 4 g, Phosphorus 1 mg, Potassium (K) 78mg, Sodium (Na) 54mg, Protein 14g

# Mini Burgers

Prep time:5 minutes, Cook time:20 minutes, Servings:2

**Ingredients:**

- ¼ cup arugula
- 1 tsp. black pepper
- 1 egg white
- 2 hamburger buns
- 5 oz. lean grass-fed ground beef
- 1 tsp. paprika
- 1 chopped green onion

**Preparation:**

1. Preheat the broiler/grill to medium-high heat.
2. Mix the ground beef with the herbs, egg white, spices and chopped green onion.
3. Use your hands to form 2 patties (about 1 inch thick).
4. Add to an oven-proof baking tray and broil for 15 minutes or until meat is thoroughly cooked through. (Use a knife to insert into the center - the juices should run clear).
5. Slice your burger buns and stack with the burger and arugula.

**Nutritional information:**

Calories 227, Protein 17 g, Carbs 23 g, Fat 7 g, Sodium (Na) 295 mg, Potassium (K) 78 mg, Phosphorus 193 mg

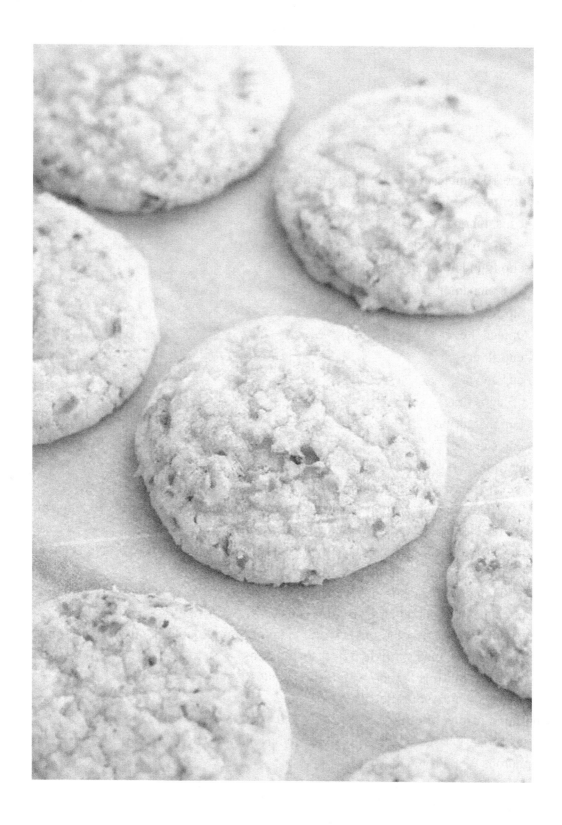

# Desserts

## Raspberry Muffins

Prep time:10 minutes, Cook time:20 minutes, Servings:10

**Ingredients:**

- 2 tbsps. margarine
- 1 ½ tsps. baking soda
- ½ cup liquid non-dairy creamer
- 2 tsps. cinnamon
- 1 cup fresh raspberries
- 1 Omega-3 egg
- ¼ cup flour
- ½ cup stevia
- 1 1/3 cups flour
- ¼ cup margarine
- ¼ cup stevia

**Preparation:**

1. Preheat your oven to a temperature of 375°F.
2. Line 16 muffin cups with paper liners; then combine about 1 and 1/3 cups of flour with the baking soda in a small bowl and stir in the raspberries
3. In a separate medium bowl; beat the ¼ cup of margarine with the brown sugar and the egg and blender very well
4. Add in the flour and stir until your mixture becomes smooth
5. Spoon the batter in about 16 muffin cups
6. In another bowl, mix the stevia with ¼ cup of flour, 2 tablespoons of margarine and the cinnamon; then sprinkle it over the muffins
7. Bake your muffins for about 15 to 18 minutes
8. Serve and enjoy your muffins!

**Nutritional information:**

Calories 156.2, Fat 10g, Carbs 13g, Potassium (K) 56mg, Sodium (Na) 111mg, Phosphorous 69g, Protein 3g

# Kidney-friendly Unsalted Pretzels

Prep time:15 minutes, Cook time:15 minutes, Servings:12

**Ingredients:**

- 1 tbsp. sesame seeds
- ¾ cup warm water
- 2 cups flour
- 1 tbsp. stevia
- 1 pack dry yeast
- 2 tbsps. almond milk

**Preparation:**

1. Mix the dry yeast with warm water; then add in the stevia and beat in the flour
2. Knead your dough until it becomes smooth for about 10 minutes
3. Place the dough over a floured surface and divide it into about 12 pieces
4. Roll the pieces into ropes of about 12 inches each
5. Shape each dough rope into the form of a pretzel; then place it over a greased baking sheet and brush it with milk
6. Sprinkle the sesame seeds; then bake your pretzels at a temperature of about 425° F for about 12 to 15 minutes
7. Let the pretzels cool for about 5 minutes
8. Serve and enjoy!

**Nutritional information:**

Calories 142, Fat 8g, Carbs 13g, Potassium (K) 61mg, Sodium (Na) 3mg, Phosphorous 48g, Protein 3.5g

# Vanilla Custard

Prep time:5 minutes, Cook time:30 minutes, Servings:3

## Ingredients:

- Artificial sweetener
- 1 large vegan egg
- 1/8 tsp. vanilla
- 1/8 tsp. nutmeg
- ½ cup low-fat milk
- 2 tbsps. stevia

## Preparation:

1. Scald the milk then let it cool slightly.
2. Break the egg into a small bowl and beat it with the nutmeg
3. Add the scalded milk, the vanilla and the sweetener to taste; then mix very well
4. Place the bowl in a baking pan filled with ½ deep of water and bake for about 30 minutes at a temperature of about 325° F
5. Serve and enjoy your custard!

## Nutritional information:

Calories 167.3, Fat 9g, Carbs 11g, Potassium (K) 249mg, Sodium (Na) 124mg, Phosphorous 205g, Protein 10g

# Almond Cookies

Prep time:7 minutes, Cook time:10 minutes, Servings:10

**Ingredients:**

- 1 tsp. almond extract
- 1 cup stevia
- 1 tsp. baking soda
- 1 vegan egg
- 1 cup softened margarine
- 3 cups white flour

**Preparation:**

1. Cream the margarine in a bowl; then add the stevia to it and beat very well
2. Sift your dry ingredients and add it to the creamed mixture
3. Add in the almond extract and mix very well.
4. Roll the dough into balls of about ¾ inches in diameter.
5. Make a small hole in each of the cookies and bake for about 12 minutes at a temperature of 400° F
6. Let the cookies cool for about 10 minutes
7. Serve and enjoy your dessert!

**Nutritional information:**

Calories 88, Fat 5g, Carbs 8g, Potassium (K) 28mg, Sodium (Na) 99mg, Phosphorous 30g, Protein 2.3g

# Chocolate Chip Cookies

Prep time:7 minutes, Cook time:10 minutes, Servings:10

**Ingredients:**

- ½ cup semi-sweet chocolate chips
- ½ tsp. baking soda
- ½ tsp. vanilla
- ¼ tsp. salt
- 1 beaten vegan egg
- 1 cup flour
- ½ cup margarine
- 4 tsps. stevia

**Preparation:**

1. Sift your dry ingredients all together
2. Cream the margarine; the stevia, the vanilla and the egg and whisk very well
3. Add flour mixture and beat again
4. Stir in the chocolate chips; then drop teaspoonfuls of the mixture over a greased baking sheet
5. Bake your cookies for about 10 minutes at a temperature of 375° F
6. Let your cookies cool for 5 minutes
7. Serve and enjoy your chocolate chip cookies!

**Nutritional information:**

Calories 106.2, Fat 7g, Carbs 8.9g, Potassium (K) 28mg, Sodium (Na) 98mg, Phosphorous 19g, Protein 1.5g

# Fruit Compote

Prep time:5 minutes, Cook time:30 minutes, Servings:3

## Ingredients:

- 28 oz. pineapple chunks
- 28 oz. pear slices

## For the cherry pie filling:

- ¼ cup melted margarine
- 2 cups crushed almond flakes

## Preparation:

1. Wash and drain your fruits very well; then grease a baking pan with cooking spray
2. Cut your fruits into slices; then arrange the fruit slices in the bottom of your baking pan
3. Crush the Grease a 9 x 13-inch pan and layer fruit, ending with pie filling.
4. Crush the almond flakes; then mix it with the margarine and sprinkle it over the fruits
5. Bake your pie for about 30 minutes at a temperature of 350°F
6. Serve and enjoy your dessert!

## Nutritional information:

Calories 135.2, Fats 10g, Carbs 8.5g, Potassium (K) 286mg, Sodium (Na) 115mg, Phosphorous 32g, Protein 2.5g

# Puffed Cereal Bars

Prep time:5 minutes, Cook time:10 minutes, Servings:10

## Ingredients:

- 8 cups puffed rice cereal
- 1 ½ cups stevia
- 1/3 cup margarine
- 1 tsp. maple extract

## Preparation:

1. In a large saucepan and over medium high heat, melt the margarine; then stir in the stevia, the maple extract and let boil for about 7 to 10 minutes
2. Stir in the puffed rice cereal; then let the mixture cool for about 5 minutes
3. Press the mixture into a greased baking pan and let chill for about 15 minutes
4. Cut into about 20 bars
5. Serve and enjoy your dessert!

## Nutritional information:

Calories 111, Fat 7.9g, Carbs 6.4g, Potassium (K) 10mg, Sodium (Na) 26mg, Phosphorous 15g, Protein 3g

# Strawberry Ice-cream

Prep time:5 minutes, Cook time:5 minutes, Servings:3

**Ingredients:**

- ½ cup stevia
- 1 tbsp. lemon juice
- ¾ cup non-dairy coffee creamer
- 10-oz unsweetened strawberries
- 1 cup crushed ice

**Preparation:**

1. Thaw the strawberries until it starts breaking up into chunks
2. Blend your ingredients until it becomes smooth
3. Pour your mixture into a dish
4. Freeze the ice cream in the dish for about 1 hour
5. Serve and enjoy your dessert!

**Nutritional information:**

Calories 94.4, Fat 6g, Carbs 8.3g, Potassium (K) 108mg, Sodium (Na) 25mg, Phosphorous 25g, Protein 1.3g

# Appendix: Measurements and Conversions

## Volume

| Imperial | Metric | | Imperial | Metric |
|---|---|---|---|---|
| 1 tbsp | 15ml | | 1 pint | 570 ml |
| 2 fl oz | 55 ml | | 1 ¼ pints | 725 ml |
| 3 fl oz | 75 ml | | 1 ¾ pints | 1 litre |
| 5 fl oz (¼ pint) | 150 ml | | 2 pints | 1.2 litres |
| 10 fl oz (½ pint) | 275 ml | | 2½ pints | 1.5 litres |
| | | | 4 pints | 2.25 litres |

## Weight

| Imperial | Metric | | Imperial | Metric | | Imperial | Metric |
|---|---|---|---|---|---|---|---|
| ½ oz | 10 g | | 4 oz | 110 g | | 10 oz | 275 g |
| ¾ oz | 20 g | | 4½ oz | 125 g | | 12 oz | 350 g |
| 1 oz | 25 g | | 5 oz | 150 g | | 1 lb | 450 g |
| 1½ oz | 40 g | | 6 oz | 175 g | | 1 lb 8 oz | 700 g |
| 2 oz | 50 g | | 7 oz | 200 g | | 2 lb | 900 g |
| 2½ oz | 60 g | | 8 oz | 225 g | | 3 lb | 1.35 kg |
| 3 oz | 75 g | | 9 oz | 250 g | | | |

# Metric Cups Conversion

| Cups | Imperial | Metric |
|------|----------|--------|
| 1 cup flour | 5oz | 150g |
| 1 cup caster or granulated sugar | 8oz | 225g |
| 1 cup soft brown sugar | 6oz | 175g |
| 1 cup soft butter/margarine | 8oz | 225g |
| 1 cup sultanas/raisins | 7oz | 200g |
| 1 cup currants | 5oz | 150g |
| 1 cup ground almonds | 4oz | 110g |
| 1 cup oats | 4oz | 110g |
| 1 cup golden syrup/honey | 12oz | 350g |
| 1 cup uncooked rice | 7oz | 200g |
| 1 cup grated cheese | 4oz | 110g |
| 1 stick butter | 4oz | 110g |
| ¼ cup liquid (water, milk, oil etc) | 4 tablespoons | 60ml |
| ½ cup liquid (water, milk, oil etc) | ¼ pint | 125ml |
| 1 cup liquid (water, milk, oil etc) | ½ pint | 250ml |

# Oven Temperatures

| Gas Mark | Fahrenheit | Celsius | Gas Mark | Fahrenheit | Celsius |
|----------|-----------|---------|----------|-----------|---------|
| 1/4 | 225 | 110 | 4 | 350 | 180 |
| 1/2 | 250 | 130 | 5 | 375 | 190 |
| 1 | 275 | 140 | 6 | 400 | 200 |
| 2 | 300 | 150 | 7 | 425 | 220 |
| 3 | 325 | 170 | 8 | 450 | 230 |
|  |  |  | 9 | 475 | 240 |

# Oven temperatures

| Gas Mark | Fahrenheit | Celsius | | Gas Mark | Fahrenheit | Celsius |
|----------|------------|---------|---|----------|------------|---------|
| 1/4 | 225 | 110 | | 4 | 350 | 180 |
| 1/2 | 250 | 130 | | 5 | 375 | 190 |
| 1 | 275 | 140 | | 6 | 400 | 200 |
| 2 | 300 | 150 | | 7 | 425 | 220 |
| 3 | 325 | 170 | | 8 | 450 | 230 |
| | | | | 9 | 475 | 240 |

# Weight

| Imperial | Metric | | Imperial | Metric |
|----------|--------|---|----------|--------|
| ½ oz | 10 g | | 6 oz | 175 g |
| ¾ oz | 20 g | | 7 oz | 200 g |
| 1 oz | 25 g | | 8 oz | 225 g |
| 1½ oz | 40 g | | 9 oz | 250 g |
| 2 oz | 50 g | | 10 oz | 275 g |
| 2½ oz | 60 g | | 12 oz | 350 g |
| 3 oz | 75 g | | 1 lb | 450 g |
| 4 oz | 110 g | | 1 lb 8 oz | 700 g |
| 4½ oz | 125 g | | 2 lb | 900 g |
| 5 oz | 150 g | | 3 lb | 1.35 kg |

# Conclusion

Following a Renal Diet means following a diet that may be less taxing on your kidneys and therefore may slow the development of kidney disease. While your doctor may ask you to limit your sodium intake, choose high-quality protein sources and potentially limit your potassium intake, with the recipes contained in this book you can still enjoy delicious meals and meet your specific health goals.

You should also make sure that these practices become a habit for you and you will definitely start to notice a positive change in your overall health!

Made in the USA
Coppell, TX
15 February 2020